Touching the Essentials

Touching the Essentials

May Shaked and Itai Rossman

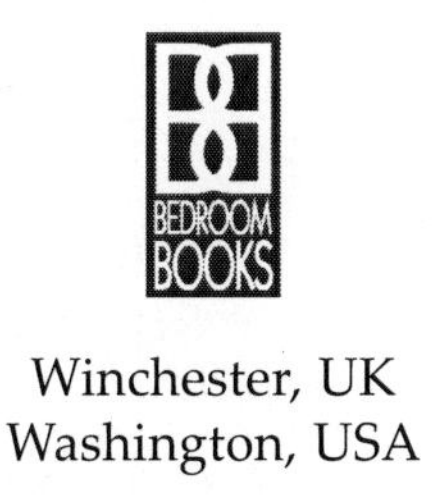

Winchester, UK
Washington, USA

First published by Bedroom Books, 2015
Bedroom Books is an imprint of John Hunt Publishing Ltd., Laurel House, Station Approach, Alresford, Hants, SO24 9JH, UK
office1@jhpbooks.net
www.johnhuntpublishing.com
www.bedroom-books.com

For distributor details and how to order please visit the 'Ordering' section on our website.

ISBN: 978 1 78099 321 8

A CIP catalogue record for this book is available from the British Library.

Design: Stuart Davies

Printed in the USA by Edwards Brothers Malloy

CONTENTS

Disclaimer

This book was written based on experience and knowledge accumulated from both personal knowledge and the development of ancient techniques and methods. Every technique may not be suitable for every individual, and there are some that may cause physical harm.

In any event, this book is not meant to be a replacement for individual consultation with a psychologist, sexologist or medical professional; the authors are not responsible for any outcome resulting from the use of concepts found in this book.

A sort of Introduction

Once upon a time

On one clear day, my partner and I decided to write a guide for better, enhanced sex. Why, you ask? You'll understand soon. My name is May, and 26 years ago, I burst into the world screaming. I grew up in the suburbs of Northern Israel, finished high school, served an average and emotionless period in the Israeli army. And, after finishing my two years of mandatory service, I traveled to the Far East – much like many others Israelis do after the army.

I first had sex during high school. I have to admit that the experience left me with a bad taste in my mouth… I just couldn't understand what the commotion was about. And why sex is made into such a 'big deal.'

'That's it?' I thought, 'All that fuss over this?'

It wasn't my poor partner's fault. Even though he was two years older than me, he didn't have much more experience than I did. And so, it ended as soon as it started: Before I could even say 'Abracadabra,' I was supposed to have already finished my first incredible orgasm, and within the nanosecond that one of us did experience it…

Before finishing my army service, I added a few more 'embarrassing situations' to my collection of sexual experiences. Finally, I was convinced that bells only ring in church and stars can be only seen while looking through a telescope.

During my tour in the Far East, I got 'up close and personal' with a number of young men from different places around the world (Denmark, United States, England, etc). For the first time in my life, I felt like I learned a thing or two about sex: I finally understood that it is possible to enjoy sexual intercourse, even a few times in the same night.

It turns out that there is a good reason for the mass

production of condoms...

I met Itai, my partner both in life and in the writing of this book, at the end of the trip.

We met by chance at one of the hotels on Khao San Road in Bankok, Thailand. The second I noticed the handsome Israeli man who was older than me by more than a few years, my heart started pounding so loudly that I thought it could be heard from far away...

But, apparently I was the only one to hear my heart beating, because Itai sent no sign of returning my interest. A week later, we met for the second time. We were on our way to the Islands, and this time, I mustered up some courage and deliberately sat next to him, hoping that a 12-hour trip would make him talk to me.

When we finally started talking, I found out that Itai was from Tel Aviv, the graduate of an elite army combat unit, and that he was about to finish a BA in Communications. According to him, he'd decided to travel to the Far East to 'cut himself off' from everything.

Needless to say, by the end of the trip we had rented a room together and caved to the lust that had begun burning between us...

We will never forget that first night: Our sex was simply incredible. We tried everything we had managed to learn from our fully receptive partners on each other, and of course, also added a few new discoveries of our own...

At the end of a romantic month on the Thai Islands, we decided to carry out an in-depth investigation on the subject of sex. We flew to India and went to different ashrams in order to learn Eastern doctrine and theory.

This was just the beginning of our journey. We stayed with Chinese teachers, we visited Scandinavia, Europe, the United States, and we tried every technique, position and local trend while it was 'fresh.'

When we understood that the scope of our accumulated knowledge and experience was close to that of the best sexologists, we knew that had to share this message with all those people who weren't able to go to around the world looking for different dogmas and learning firsthand about the secrets of sex customary outside of Israel.

From that, the book that we wrote pulls together the best pieces of information that we acquired across the ocean. While it is personal and individual, it also refers to everyone: women, men, young people, adults, those with experience, and those at the very beginning of their 'professional' path…

This book does not pretend to contain every issue related to sex, like for example, fetishes (which are all about personal taste), kissing, stroking the chest, tickling the back, etc. (because we believe that these abilities come naturally to each of us.). Instead, it includes the more central and important elements that will help you go from being mediocre – or even good – lovers to being excellent lovers, the kind that your partner's friends want to meet.

To keep from exhausting you with an unlimited amount of information or review things you surely know already, we chose to present just the main, unique and most important aspects of each topic.

For all the curious boys and girls amongst you: Itai and I returned to Israel, settled down in a rustic dream house, and continue to be a 'charming, loving couple' – that's what everyone says about us anyway.

We've already begun thinking seriously about our next book. But, in the meantime, we hope you enjoy this book, along with the self-development and exciting experiences toward which it will lead you.

Enjoy!

May and Itai

Nice to meet you

Some names it's important to remember in this book

So that we won't sound too scientific or callous, we chose nicknames to represent the main actors – the active people and limbs in this story.

Please welcome them:

Jessica

The sexy star of the play is you, girl. Trust me, your partner also thinks the resemblance between you two is not in any way accidental; otherwise you wouldn't have gotten to this point…

Rabbit

Yeah, man, we gave you a name with expectations. But, we have a feeling that it suits you perfectly. After all, *Jessica* deserves nothing less…

Angelina

The delicate beauty that lives between your legs, *Jessica*. Your *Rabbit's* soul mate and the precious treasure destined to receive royal treatment. In other books, she is called 'the vulva.'

Fabio

Rabbit's 'secret weapon' who is just waiting to conquer *Angelina*'s magical kingdom. He also likes toys and pampering, and just between us – he really deserves it. In other classes, he is known as the 'penis.'

And now, after we've all been introduced, we can begin…

Chapter 1

Clearing the Air: Personal hygiene and appearance

In order to turn the intimate 'summit' into an enjoyable, sensual and exciting experience, it is important to pay attention to a number of hygiene rules that will 'clear the air.' If you don't pay attention to these minor details, Karius' and Bactus' cousins, 'The Stickies,' will likely be invited to your private party, which will cause 'Slow,' who is tight with your partner to seem like a cautious Secret Service invasion – covered with a gas mask as they enter an area infected with tuberculosis. If you don't want sex to end before it begins, you should be considerate of the leading players on this 'athletic field' – some of whom are more famous than others.

Polishing Wax

The first people on the 'Clean the Air' ladder are, of course, '**Mister Clean**' and '**Miss Aroma**' – who set the main tone for any contact between two people, and especially between those intending to 'take down the dividers' and get thoroughly acquainted with one another's secret hiding places.

A few little soap bubbles

If you want to avoid imposing 'your tough day' onto the shoulder of your excited partner, make sure to shower before every sexual interaction. Also, be sure to foam up at least twice so that the crotch area and genitals smell nice before the imminent 'liquid transfer.' Our suggestion, to both the women and men out there, is to do a '**two-stage wash**' in the lively 'activity' area. Shampoo of any type will give you the most thorough lathering.

'Two-stage washing' is as simple as it sounds:

a Wet the area with water.
b Lather up using shampoo.
c Rinse again with water.
d Lather up a second time with shampoo.
e Final rinsing with water.

Training the rebellious

If you girls have given up because of frequent rinsing and the 'fragrance' that sneaks out from between your legs, let me tell you about an amazingly effective product that gets rid of acidity from the genitals and turns your rebellious *Angelina* into an especially clean and aromatic maiden. It is called intimate cleanser (or feminine wash). This patented invention makes 'fragranced intruders' evaporate almost completely from our Norwegian princess. A single use of this blessed product is worth four intensive showers with regular soap. So, basically, we enable noble *Angelina* to enjoy maximum sterilization with minimum effort.

Many companies produce the intimate soap – some of them are good, others are better; we will leave it up to you, girls of the beautiful gender, to trial and error until you find the product that best and most effectively works for you.

Remember

'Scrubbing and polishing' *Angelina* will encourage your partner to wholeheartedly take her in, strum on her with his beloved fingers and give her 'French kisses' with his skilled tongue.

Important note

Frequent, long-term use of the intimate cleanser is not healthy. So, it is not recommended to 'condition' *Angelina* with it for a long period of time. However, to prevent any sudden hesitation by your enthusiastic partner from licking your 'sweet honey,' make sure to use it before the 'summit.'

The Scent Department

The secondary actors in this significant department are: perfume, deodorant, aftershave (for men), etc. They are important and influential – both before sex and in everyday life. We highly recommend that both genders make frequent and habitual use of them. The goal is to maintain basic hygiene, smell good and allow other people to have a conversation with you through their mouth and not from afar, while using a 'walkie-talkie'.

These things are also relevant (and essential) before sex. The use of each of these secondary actors is particularly critical, as we haven't yet heard of an alternative for having intimate contact through a remote control (unless you're a virtual sex fiend, but you didn't purchase this book for that reason...).

Fisherman's Syndrome

In order to separate us from the animals with flippers and gills, a dandruff problem should be dealt with.

Dandruff is dry skin that falls off of the scalp, and is likely to cover your head with a very unappealing rash.

To deal with a light dandruff problem, you can (and should) use a shampoo that prevents dandruff (of which many exist); in more severe cases, you should visit a dermatologist.

Pooh Bear and the Honeycomb

If there is anything that can discourage a partner, it is excess dirt in the ears. As they come to give you 'culinary treatment' in the ear, they will be shocked to discover bitter residue in the place of a nice, soft piece of meat. Therefore, before the 'summit,' we highly recommend making sure to clean your ears.

Sweat is thick with water

Perspiration is a very sensitive stethoscope able to identify the type of food you ate today, or even yesterday. Foods with garlic, onion, or curry affect your sweat and will cause your bodies to emit a strong and suffocating odor exactly at the critical moment.

So, we highly recommend that you avoid eating these ingredients the day before the wild dance – as much as possible. Despite praise garlic has won from conventional medicine, our research proves that its ability to chase away a partner is more effective than its ability to chase off bacteria…

Drunk, and not from wine or the 'Space Odyssey'

After waking up or eating something spicy, your mouth cavity will often be enveloped with a heavy odor that carries distances. Therefore, in addition to a meticulous mouth cleansing, take a piece of advice from your amigo and chew a piece of gum about ten minutes before your important date and about fifteen minutes before the 'summit.'

For those that wake up together or enjoy an entire day as a team (since the mouth begins to accumulate unpleasant smells during the evening hours), we recommend picking up the cup of juice awaiting you by the bedside and reducing the mouth odor before a much awaited kiss...

In acute cases, when the juice's smell has died out, you can begin to wander with your mouth toward other areas of your partner's body, which may 'sniff' a bit, but lack a sense of smell…

Important note

Chronic odor is defined as a medical problem. Those suffering from it should go to the Ear, Nose & Throat (ENT) Doctor to get quick, effective treatment.

Did you know?

Eating parsley and drinking a lot of water help to get rid of unpleasant mouth odors.

Lubrication Oil (Lube)

A no-less critical stage in preparing for the upcoming 'Summit' deals with hygiene and softening the 'coarse sands' of the 'conquered' territory. Rough skin is not pleasant to touch, and so, it is important to soften it.

The palm of your hand

Hygiene – Keep your hands clean (fingernails too, of course). This is important both for hygiene and health. After all, the hands tend to enter into all kinds of deep and sensitive tunnels, and friendly bacteria are not welcome in the 'hallowed halls.'

Softening – Touching with hands is no less important than their cleanliness. Everyone agrees that a soft, smooth touch is more attractive than the feeling of being stroked with sandpaper. Therefore, men and women, if soft, fragrant hands are your heart's desire, then make sure to apply some nice, perfumed hand cream to them.

Feet

Hygiene – In every issue related to hygiene maintenance, feet are without a doubt a particularly problematic area. All day long, they are squashed into a sealed furnace filled with sweat and bacteria, and, if we're talking about sneakers, the festival is really big. Damp toes accrue strong smells that are able to knock out even anosmics (people with no sense of smell). From there all the way to your departing handshake – under the assumption that you've followed our instructions in the previous section – we'll take a short cut.

So, wash your feet really well before the 'summit,' especially one that may include paw pleasure with slow, sensual licking. Remember: 'Cheese' and fungus are best left for pizza and not your partner…

Softening – Spreading an aromatic body lotion or foot cream on your feet will help to soften the skin (which is sometimes course and rough) and will help bring 'Miss Aroma' into the picture. The cream keeps the foot pleasant and smelling good, absorbs the odor for a long time, and enables creative and pleasure-inducing use of the foot throughout the 'athletic act'...

Did you know?

The largest quantity of bacteria in the body are on the feet – more than are located in the mouth or any other part of the body.

Lips

Just like every other part of the body, the lips also need to be soft. For that reason, lipstick is the favorite invention of many women. Still, while it does its devoted work in adding color and softening the lips, many men also find their partners to be beautiful without it, and even prefer to kiss their lips without the oily mediator that stains their faces and leaves an aftertaste.

So ladies, your call!

You can certainly use your soft and glittery friend, but take into account that some partners might perceive it as a mortal enemy...

Body work and coloring

We've finally arrived at the last stage of preparations for the intimate 'summit.'

At this stage you are almost ready for the big moment, with the exception of a few significant details that separate the human race at present from the monkeys of earlier eras.

'Pruning' the genitals

Ladies and gentlemen! If you feel like preserving the trees and forests, join Greenpeace. But, in every aspect of body esthetics, your genitalia are not a thick forest.

Below you will find a few trimming methods that will not damage a flower or stem, but will maintain their beauty...

Types of 'pruning':

It is important to clarify that part of this is targeted at men and women together, since a sterile environment for the stalk is no less important than one for the flower. In both cases, long hair, which tends to accumulate smell, will chase away any nearby butterfly.

As you can see on any website or sex magazine, there are an unlimited number of haircuts – moderate, fashionable or conservative, and you can easily modernize with the latest 'pruning fad,' in all of its shapes and colors. But, the goal now is to give you simple, preliminary tools to turn pruning work into a 'walk in the park' instead of an attempt to level a road inside the tangled jungle.

For the purpose of simplifying the explanation, we'll separate pubic hair into three sections:

The courtyard

The part above the genitals ('esthetic pruning'):

In this region, it is very important to trim the pubic hair and to keep a well-maintained and nice-looking appearance. After all, you don't want it to be wild and neglected like Sleeping Beauty's palace, which had to 'dry out' for hundreds of years before the knight arrived…

Women: We suggest that you trim the 'yard hair' as short as possible. Make sure it isn't too sharp – 'a porcupine haircut' is likely to be prickly and unpleasant for your partner. Another option is to shave the 'yard hair' off completely, and by doing so, increasing *Angelina's* hygiene and attracting to her men that like forest clearings.

Remember: A triangular growth of hair is reasonable – it isn't a pasture, but a small piece of garden.

Men: There is no doubt that cropped pubic hair is the fashion statement of the future. In the meantime, we suggest you shorten it as much as possible, so that the tongue going down to the depths of your stalk won't lick weeds as well... An obvious advantage (on the eye): If you get rid of the tangled camouflage, the barrel of your cannon looks much larger.

'The Main Gate'

The part on the sides and at the opening of the genitals ('practical pruning'): Cutting/shaving in this area is significant for two main reasons:

1. Smell: Both men and women sweat a lot in this unventilated area. Long, wild 'bushes of hair' accumulate smell and stickiness.
2. Through the forest you can't see the bears: Long hair is likely to invade your partner's mouth. So, instead of being blinded by the buried treasure and giving it the desired treatment, your partner will be busy spitting out wandering hairs, picking at their mouth and 'clearing a path'...

It is hard for us to believe that this is how you imagined the fertilization of your flower/stalk.

This region can also be treated in one of two ways:

- Shortening it significantly, but not so much that the act of going down on you will turn into an experience of wading through a thorn field.
- The 'Michael Jordan' shave – smooth like the infamous basketball idol's bald head.

This has both advantages and disadvantages:

- For: The smooth haircut completely conceals unpleasant odors.
- Against: After the shaving, the area where hair grows fills with red dots. There are men who do not find this red rash to be particularly attractive.

'The King's Path'

It begins just behind the genitals and continues all the way through to the anus.

Men: If you want your partners to 'completely devote themselves' to the area (a more in-depth description is in the 'Kitchenette' chapter) you should treat this with the utmost seriousness.

If you choose the 'Trimming Route' – go for it, but make sure that the thorns don't scratch the soft, delicate skin on your amazing partner's face... also, be careful while doing it. It's a dead zone (in terms of your field of vision), and we wouldn't want to damage it or anything nearby.

The most highly recommended way to a 'safe cut' is with an electronic shaver for nose and ear hairs (further explanation for how to use this machine can be found later in the chapter).

Women: The clear, unequivocal rules of esthetics do not permit hair to exist in the area between *Angelina* and the anus, including on the anus itself.

So what can you do?

Shave, wax, pluck, do whatever you want, on the condition that this area shines and smells like the neighbor's flower planters.

For those that have trouble with the pruning work, there are expert hairdressers that do it. They will be happy to advise you on up-to-date trimming trends and give your *Angelina* a fashionable, representative, good 'look.'

For those of you interested in turning pruning work into an intimate, unique experience with a partner, I suggest increasing the sexual tension with your partner by shaving *Angelina* in a different way each time. For example, do it with the Nike symbol, another time dye it a bright green (as they say: your grass is greener), another time let it grow out fully, or show it totally exposed in its full naked glory, and there are many other original shapes.

Remember

The Courtyard, including the Main Gate, is your private territory and you are welcome to do anything with it that enters your wild imagination.

Important Note

Pruning is likely to cause red rashes or pimples on those with sensitive skin. Therefore, in order to allow the skin irritation to disappear, we recommend you cut the 'royal Norwegian girls' a few days before the long-awaited moment.

Did you know?

The trend of pruning pubic hair began to gain momentum only in the 1990s, and since then has been 'blooming'.

Tips for the new gardener

For those of you interested in a 'Michael Jordan' haircut, but having trouble finding a hairdresser to give *Angelina* the desired treatment, or those interested in doing the work with their own hands, I have compiled a few 'slicing' instructions for doing the job:

a If you have long, impressive tresses, first use a pair of scissors or a haircutting device. This 'shortening' activity will make the job of shaving easier for you, and will enable clean, precise pruning.
b After shortening it, soften the 'Fortress Hair' with soap,

shampoo or conditioner, and prepare it for the next stage.

c After you've removed the conditioning material and have washed the area with water, wipe *Angelina* dry and cover her with shaving gel. Rub the gel on the hair until you've achieve the desired softness.

d Important Note: Women with delicate skin are advised to choose a gel for sensitive skin that prevents irritations and rashes.

e Before the pruning work itself, take a new, high quality razor, which makes the shaving easier and will prevent pimples and skin irritations. It is also very important that you make every effort to keep the shaving gel from finding its way into the vagina – this is not healthy and is also likely to burn.

f At the end of the pruning work, wash the area with water and make sure that you didn't miss any key points in *Angelina's* haircut. If you find rebellious branches that disrupt the harmony of the forest, re-spread the gel and complete your work.

g At the end of the haircut, it is good to spread moisturizing cream on sexy *Angelina* in order assist the skin and to prevent unwanted irritations.

Girls, you should be ready for the fact that *Angelina* is likely to rebel against initial haircuts and develop irritations and rashes. However, the longer you continue doing pruning work, the phenomenon will decrease and the rebellious princess will learn to smile gratefully. Good luck!

Trimming the entire lawn

In addition to 'hot regions' – the areas owned by *Fabio* and *Angelina* – there are other places on the body that need shaving or plucking to prevent the talked-about 'Baboon Affect.'

Men – Besides the fact that you're more hairy by nature, it is a well-known phenomenon that men over the age of thirty go through a number of physiological ups and downs: the metabolism slows down (and causes an increase in weight), and the rate of hair growth increases in certain areas of the body.

Ladies – An unfortunate, but existing, fact is that society is less forgiving to women with hair in different places on the body than it is to men. And so, you should pluck or shave in other places.

Below are a few places of note for both sexes that will help you to get through the meeting with the other sex 'smoothly.'

Mustache/beard

Guy – Besides the fact that the goatee and Hitler mustache trends died somewhere in the 70s, along with disco, we highly recommend shaving your mustache and beard before an intimate encounter. Your partner will certainly prefer that you scratch her body in other places, and not on her soft face or Norwegian princess.

Girl – In your case as well, the 'Dictator Effect' doesn't really do the job, and we wholeheartedly suggest you pluck facial hair, including a mustache. Note that peroxide is not always effective, as it can cause the hair to grow and reproduce faster than normal.

Hair on Arms and Hands

Men – While there are women who are opposed to fur-covered hands, the issue is up to your personal judgment. Always remember that there are those who see it as a symbol of masculinity and their dream is to be the Jane to your Tarzan.

Women – If we're discussing a thick shell of hair, we suggest removing it. I've never heard of men who dream of being the Jane to their female Tarzan...

Hair on legs and Feet

Men – Here too, the extreme difference in society's treatment of the two genders pops up. Men (mostly in the past year, with the retro to furriness), are welcome to grow hair on their legs. In most cases, it is even considered to be desirable and attractive.

Women – It is acceptable that women (except particularly fervent feminists) pluck or shave the hair on their legs and feet, in order to distinguish their soft, smooth legs from men's rough, wild bodies.

Stomach Hair

Men – Just as in the paragraph above, nature endowed most men with thick hair on the stomach. Men are split on this issue: there are those that make sure to pull out the thick forest with waxing or laser hair removal, and not so that we can see what their belly-button looks like…

Women – If fate played its role and your stomach is a bit 'active' in this field, it's best if you remove the rebellious hairs with waxing or try laser treatment – leave the virgin forests to the men.

Back Hair

Men – A thin lawn will be welcomed by most women. But parsley curls are a different story and that depends on you, your partner and her personal taste.

Women – In your case, to my dismay, even a thin lawn is not acceptable. This may not bother you during the 'summit,' but if you are interested in a sensual massage, the hairs are likely to place a 'live wire' between you and your partner.

Chest/Nipple Hair

Men – With a few lucky exceptions, most men grow a vegetable garden there. For some of you it blossoms, whereas for others it specializes in miniature growths. Most men 'go with nature' and don't see any harm in this; others are influenced by movie stars and remove the hair by waxing or shaving.

Women – Hair around the nipple region is a very frequent

thing, but if it is more than just a stray hair, we suggest you pluck using tweezers.

Armpits

Men – Leave the magnificent hair as is. Just please, make sure to keep it fresh and clean. Never, no matter what, use deodorant when your armpit is sweaty. This creates a bad mix of smells.

Women – We highly recommend shaving the area or removing the hair by waxing regularly. Armpit hair is not esthetically pleasing, produces murky waves of bad odors and looks like a habitat for reptiles and their comrades from the animal kingdom.

Ears/Nose

Men – This phenomenon is unique to you, most particularly upon your arrival at the age of thirty. Suddenly, your ears are reminiscent of baby wolves and the edge of your nostrils look like a dark cave. For these issues there is a simple and quick solution: All you have to do is shave or cut the undesired hairs with a special device for cutting nose and ear hairs. This machine (around 6 inches long and shaped like a stick, enabling it to fit into deep, narrow places) can be found in every electronics store and even at a cheap price. It is very effective and not dangerous to use at all.

So, go on your way and conquer the objective 'by the hair'!

Lastly, but not always so pleasant...

The last small detail in 'conquering the form' is clipping nails. Nails are a subject of personal taste, both among men and women. Therefore, before you 'pull out your nails,' allow me to clarify the issue and turn your attention to a few of the less pleasant aspects of long, sharp nails.

Men – Long nails are likely to be full of sex appeal in your eyes, but during the 'summit,' your excited fingers are likely to scratch your partner in the 'holy of holies' and maybe even hurt her. It is hard for me to see her reacting to the affair in a particularly sexy manner...

Therefore, 'for safety purposes,' make sure to cut them a few days before the 'long awaited moment' – fingernails cut the day before are likely to be sharp and especially painful.

Women – I won't even pretend to try and convince you of what is more attractive – that is definitely an issue of taste. I just want to remind you that while on the one hand there are men that love to feel your nails during sex, there are also those for whom the touch of a sharp nail reminds them of a hungry tiger.

Chapter 2

Pleasant Rubbing: Masturbation

'Masturbation is making love to the person that you love most.'
Woody Allen

Whether or not he is right, it is definitely worth your while to learn the 'secrets of rubbing' – which are likely to be super applicable on rainy days, and can even help in 'mixing up' your 'tango for two' (if you're with a partner). The purpose of this chapter is to teach you how to pleasure your own 'fruit,' or that of your partner – regardless of whether it's an attractive-looking banana or a ripe red, juicy cherry.

'The Siren's Song'

Pleasuring the 'cherry' is not an easy task. First and foremost, this is because each and every woman is different, and each and every one of them likes it differently. There are 'cherries' that prefer gentle touching; others prefer strong, steady contact; some like it when you take them 'around the bush,' and the rest prefer 'the direct route.'

So, before we lay the entire 'bible' out for you, we recommend that you ask your partner about her preferred 'method.' Remove any doubt, friend; the last thing she'll think is that you're a 'nerd,' 'loser,' or virgin. At best, she'll feel like she won the lottery – her partner is not interested in just X, Y or Z, he also likes to indulge the 'gate' in front of the 'great rift'...

Remember

Showing interest in your partner's needs will arouse in her respect and appreciation for you, and not the opposite. Your

Jessica will immediately understand that you are a loving and giving *Rabbit* who is able to listen and open to talking about new things. (You are, of course, quick, multitasking *Rabbits*!).

A few rounds of shots to start with:

Before receiving the comprehensive treatment from *Rabbit*, we suggest that you women check out your tortilla on your own. The purpose is for you to be well acquainted with your own sexual genitalia and its needs before *Rabbit's* finger carries out its wicked plan. There are a few things that you should find out about your 'cherry': its preferred finger location, speed, force and the timing for increasing pressure (as in: just before orgasm, throughout, etc.).

Your purpose, *Brando*, is to mimic *Jessica's* actions, and in the future, do them even better than she does; which will certainly give her immense pleasure. We suggest having the first session (or even the first few, if you need it) 'on the wet.' Watch your *Jessica* masturbating, or even place your fingers on hers while she masturbates to receive a 'first-hand' demonstration. This will turn your partner on like you wouldn't believe and is also the best way to help you learn her favorite technique.

Important note

Before stroking the cherry 'seed' – better known as the clitoris – you need to do prep work on the surrounding site. Direct contact without advanced preparation instantly stimulates the many nerves found in that spot and is likely to jolt *Jessica*.

Let the games begin!

So what should you do?

You can start by stroking the thighs, and continuing to lightly flutter your hand over her pubic hairs (to 'get the area ready'), then begin softly stroking the outer labia and, finally, reaching the inner labia as well. This is the stage at which you can put a little bit of pressure on the guardians of the 'seed,' the outer labia. Force shouldn't be used, since this is a soft, gentle body part; however, light pinches are definitely within the range of possibility.

At this stage of the 'opening shots,' you're welcome to do anything that enters into your wild imagination (with the complete agreement of your partner, of course). Move the tip of your finger in and out of *Angelina's* 'hot oven,' graze *Fabio's* rim (the glans) back and forth over Katie's lips (labia), continue to stroke the excited 'guards,' pamper the interior 'security guards' – the inner labia, and more…

Trust *Jessica* to let you know what feels nice for her – whether by raising her pelvis, spreading her legs or by letting out increasingly strong moans of pleasure – or whatever else gets her light-headed.

The initial goal is to get the area wet (if it's not already wet from the start), and in the moment that *Angelina* fills up with juicy pleasure, slip your fingers into her smooth slope like an Olympic surfer.

In the second stage, we recommend wetting your fingers – either by nonchalantly putting them into your mouth or by allowing her to sensually suck your fingers. Now, move them gently over her breasts or take them for a romantic trip to the area behind *Angelina* and in front of the anus.

Trust me: this will get her excited until she loses control, jumping her stimulation levels up to the sky.

Important note

Saliva on its own cannot serve as a replacement for *Angelina's* natural lubricant. Using it is just to enrich the moisture already in the area, and to increase the intensity of your partner's arousal.

Method Number 1 – 'Rosh HaNikra'

General:

The idea behind this method is to climb up in *Angelina's* slope, and to find a resting spot in the clitoris region, with the purpose of teaching us – men – how to pleasure our *Jessica* and provide her with exterior treatment, as opposed to interior (which will be explained later).

The sad truth is that most of us naughty, and sometimes clumsy *Rabbits,* don't always have the ability to definitively find this tiny button – the clitoris.

Therefore, in this section, you will get a clear, thorough explanation about the location of this evasive button, how to feel it, and finally, the way to 'hit the bullseye,' even if you don't know exactly where it is.

Field orientation:

As you can see, our Norwegian princess is composed of a few different parts:

1. **Outer labia** (labia majora): They are generally covered with hair which is meant to protect them and the entire system.
2. **Inner labia** (labia minora): These sensitive lips are hidden within the external ones. When stimulated, they tend to become swollen and turn redder in color from the accumulation of blood.
3. **Clitoris**: 'The Miracle Button' is located at the meeting point of the inner labia, at *Angelina*'s upper end. It has no reproduction-related function; its sole purpose is to provide our *Jessica* with sexual pleasure. It is comprised of the clitoris (glans), and is surrounded by the clitoral hood – skin meant to prevent direct abrasion with the clitoris, and thereby protecting it. The clitoris can be exposed by

> moving the skin that covers it; but according to many women, because this is the most sensitive spot and has many nerve endings, direct stimulation is likely to irritate.

The size of a clitoris varies between 3 and 10 millimeters in a regular state.

While the clitoris is stimulated, a large amount of blood flows into it, significantly increasing its size and inflating it. It is good for you to know, little panthers, that during clitoral stimulation, it will conceal itself behind the outer labia. This not because of anything you did. That's its nature. So, when *Angelina*'s 'Miracle Button' asks for shelter under the protection of the inner 'security guards', continue what you're doing without worry – it will thank you for this later.

Remember

While pleasuring the clitoris, make sure to focus on it alone and not on other areas. This 'work' requires a lot of concentration, and any movement from the 'Miracle Button' is likely to throw *Jessica* off-course and destroy your shared magical moment.

Now, after you've gotten the general idea about the clitoris and its location in the upper area of the inner labia, you're ready to receive a useful tip: Work using two fingers together! Since the area is not very big, placing two fingers on the upper section of the inner lips will cover the entire area and ensure that you hit the 'slippery rascal.'

To those among you with experience

Only use one finger if you are 100% sure you know where *Jessica's* clitoris is. If you are arrogant and try to pleasure her with one finger without knowing its exact location, you are likely to miss it and start off on the wrong foot with the 'slippery rascal.'

FIRST THINGS FIRST

First and most important is the motion: There are an infinite number of movements that allow *Rabbit* to pleasure *Angelina's* clitoris, and you are certainly welcome to try them all. However, allow me to suggest one incredible motion that will turn pampering the 'Miracle Button' into an extraordinary experience –because of the comfort and ease the movement allows. The idea is this: You sit next to *Jessica,* who lies on her back, just slightly above *Angelina* (near the lower stomach) facing *Jessica's* feet with your back to *her* face. The goal is to work your indulgent fingers on the 'Miracle Button' in the same direction and angle that *Jessie's* fingers move when she masturbates. This way you will achieve maximum effectiveness because *Angelina* will get the treatment she's been used to for years without feeling a difference.

(For your sake, I hope that in the future she will feel a difference and will prefer your quick fingers to her own).

Another position is to sit at *Jessica's* feet,' while she lies down, with your face turned toward *Angelina* and *Jess's* legs spread around you. This way, you can pamper the 'Miracle Button' face to face and also watch your partner's face as she enjoys herself.

A third highly-recommended position combines intercourse and masturbation simultaneously, and by doing so, enhances and intensifies *Jessica's* experience. She enjoys two worlds at once.

For example: Doggy Style or the Cowgirl Position – you lie down and *Jessie* rides you while sitting straight on top of *Fabio.* Touching the clitoris at this point will speed up your partner's amazing orgasm with a priceless extra for her.

Another enhancement for the Cowgirl Position is for *Jessica* to ride you backwards – with her back turned toward your face. Put your thumb at the base of erect *Fabio,* with the tip pointed upward (so that your fingernail is directed toward your stomach) and curve the top part of your thumb in a 45 degree angle toward your face. This, my friend, is the exact spot of *Jessica's* clitoris. If she is into it – and there's almost no chance that she won't be, she'll move her hips back and forth to amplify the incredible feeling. Both the *Grand Canyon* and the 'Miracle Button' will profit from your impressive acrobatics.

Two techniques for the road:

There are two recommended ways of performing 'Rosh HaNikra' – this fantastic method to giving pleasure. You can, of course, use any technique you think of, but I'd like to share a few pieces of information that I've gathered:

The two are good together:

For this method, the work is done using two fingers – the index and middle fingers.

The idea is to put the two fingers up against the clitoris, moving without lifting them off of it. The motion can be very varied, but that also depends on each woman's personal needs. Here are a few directions to enrich your clitoral education:

- **Up and Down** – and so on and so forth. Your fingers move up, across the length of the clitoris, and then down again. Repeat.
- **To the sides** – left and right, again and again. Your fingers move on the clitoris in the motion of a pedestrian crosswalk, from right to left and then from left to right, again and again. This movement can be done for a while, and then we suggest changing to a different motion.
- **Circular motion** – Your fingers move on the clitoris in small to medium size circles (large circles do not get the job done), putting pressure on Jessica's clitoris. (This is the motion favored by most women).
- **The Suction Effect** – You can create a sucking effect on Jessica's clitoris by pulling the 'Miracle Button' with your

thumb and index finger outward and so on. You should be careful when doing this motion, since doing it too strongly can rip the 'Miracle Button' (despite its flexibility). This should be mixed with other techniques we've suggested to keep the 'festivities' exciting and not overtire the 'Miracle Button.'

Four in one:

Do this method using four fingers. The idea is to use two fingers from each hand (index and middle), hold them together tightly, and move them with moderate pressure around the clitoris.

When to push the pedal and change gears?

At the beginning of the ride down the 'Miracle Button's' slopes you should move slowly and put a small amount of pressure on the clitoris. As you continue, and *Jessica* warms up more and more, you increase the pressure and the tempo. Keep in mind, there is a limit to the pressure. Putting too much pressure will eliminate *Jessie's* enjoyment; as we mentioned earlier, the goal is not to hurt her, but instead to give her incredible pleasure. Feel your partner; don't hit the 'pedal' without paying attention. If you get the green light, continue traveling; but if the light changes, ease up and skid gently on the road.

Speed

Each woman is different from another: There are those who love a fast rhythm, others prefer a slow pace, some who enjoy a steady tempo throughout the ride, and still others (apparently the majority) who prefer an increasing pressure and tempo as they near the finish line.

Therefore, if it's your first test drive with *Jessica*, you should take the safe route and increase the rhythm and speed when leading up to the orgasm. On the other hand, if this is a regular partner, it's best to hear what she does and doesn't like 'straight from the horse's mouth.'

Important note

If your partner shows signs of finishing, continue with exactly the same movement that are you doing at that moment, and under no circumstances should you switch movements or the degree of pressure. Changes like these are likely to take your partner out of her concentration and return her (and you as well) to the starting point.

Method Number 2 – 'Me'arat HaMachpela'

Discovering America:

The internationally known name for the spot that makes *Jessica* dizzy, and without which sexual intercourse is no more than a challenging sport, is called the G-spot. We could make up stories and tell you that it's named after George Costanza, Gengis Khan or Garfield, but its origin is actually an unusually resourceful person who answers to the name Grafenberg.

And, as many of you women learned a long time ago, despite the fact that this is a hot topic on most talk shows and everywhere in modern literature, not many of your lover boys know the exact place of the evasive spot and, even if they do, they don't always know what to do with the buried treasure that's fallen into their hands. Therefore, dear men, please listen and pay attention so that this opinion held generally among women will one clear day turn into an old and forgotten myth.

General

Since the G-spot is a kind of Bermuda Triangle – everyone's heard about it but doesn't always know how to identify the exact spot – the best way to hit the bullseye is to use the 'automatic weapon' method. In other words: To 'take down' a small, tricky terrorist, we'll empty an entire cartridge over the area until we've damaged our target. Of the infinite bullets flying through the air, one will certainly arrive at our desired destination.

The Technique:

We'll begin with one finger. It's best to use the index finger (later on we can double up the digits that go into Me'arat haMachpela), and penetrate it as deeply as possible into *Angelina*. Penetrate it so that the pad is turned up (meaning, toward the Norwegian princess's stomach and not her butt). We suggest doing this as slowly as possible so that *Jessica* can adjust to the idea, be calm and relaxed.

After we've placed ourselves as deep inside as possible in the 'Me'arat HaMachpela' (approximately 5-6 centimeters), we begin to move the top two sections of the finger up; up and down. It looks like the well-known 'Come here' motion that Mrs. Smith, your elementary school teacher, loved to use when putting naughty kids in the corner.

At this point, *Rabbit*, you should already be sensing *Jessica's* reactions. If she moves with pleasure and makes contented sounds in your ear, it seems that your drill hit oil and your partner is about to become a very happy woman. From here on, we suggest continuing for a minute or so, and then moving on to the 'doubling up' stage, and adding another finger. There's also a big significance at this stage to which finger penetrates *Angelina;* it's best if you use the middle finger.

Your activity inside the 'cave' should be powerful and energetic – so that you can do the 'come here' movement fully and please *Jessica* as much as possible. However, so that you don't turn the fingering experience into a violent battle followed by blood, avoid using too much force.

Two roads lead to Rome:

In general, every woman likes you to touch her differently, and for that reason, at this point you can – and should – consult with your partner. However, when you get to the point of penetrating into the depths of the Me'arat haMachpela, it's best to come equipped with two diverse paths:

1. In life and in death, we won't separate

Put your two fingers, the index and middle fingers, next to each another, move them up and down and, together in perfect coordination do the 'come here' movement inside *Jessica's* 'cave.'

- **Advantage**: This motion is easier to do, and allows your *Rabbit* to continue in her for the duration.

2. Split forces:

Each of your fingers does the 'come here' movement separately, one after the other. The two fingers work simultaneously, but as one finger turns inward, the finger next to it turns outward, and so on.

- **Advantage**: Jessica's G-spot does not rest for a second, since the contact is consistent and ongoing.
- **Disadvantage**: This action requires more effort and is therefore more difficult for your devoted *Rabbit.*

Recommended Positions

- **'Your facial expression:'** *Jessica* lies on her back, legs spread with a pillow resting under her hips. *Rabbit* lies between her legs, facing her, and pleasures her G-spot using fast fingers.
- **'Upside down**:' *Jessica* lies on her stomach with spread legs, as *Rabbit* kneels between her legs and penetrates her G-spot. While in this position, it is important to note that the 'come here' movement is done backwards (even though the finger motions also moved with the pad in the direction of *Jessica's* stomach and her upper vagina). The disad-

vantage of this position is that it does not allow simultaneous work on 'Rosh HaNikra.'

Make a muscle:

Just like every athlete who wants remarkable achievements, we men must also know that to pick the fruits of victory, we too must practice.

Only after you've tried the amazing method to pleasure *Jessica's* G-spot will you understand how un-simple the motion is. The 'roof of the cave' creates a strong resistance, and the hand tends to get tired. And because you must try your best to avoid taking breaks in the middle – since *Jessica* is likely to lose her concentration, sink quickly and return to the starting line – your hand, which tries with all its might to find more and more power to succeed at its task, must start over from the very beginning... So, take some advice from a friend who has tested the field: Buy a tool (with a thick metal spring in the center) to strengthen the muscles in the palm of your hand and invest some time in hand exercises.

This may sound funny to you, but you'll be shocked to know that those are the exact muscles you need to develop and build up to do the continuous, skilled movement inside *Angelina's* 'Me'arat HaMachpela.'

In any case, most of you spend hours in a gym to get a bit more 'volume' in honor of the more beautiful gender, so take it one step further. Show them that it's worth their while to judge the book and not just its cover.

Did you know?

The tool for building up hand muscles also works for muscle parts activated when you massage your partner. (More about massaging your partner and the importance of doing it in Chapter 6 – Small Stuff to fill Space).

Just as I feared, I feel like it, or, Plan B:

In an emergency – when your hand yells 'Save me!' and every effort you make to keep pleasuring *Angelina* is futile, there is a back-up plan set aside for this exact dilemma . First of all, as I've already suggested before, try your best to avoid stopping the activity altogether. Second, you have the option of switching hands; but it isn't recommended as it's likely to spoil your honey's concentration.

Your faithful friend's back-up plan is: During emergency situations, you can switch the 'Come here' motion for a penetration movement, and move your two fingers in and out, exactly like skilled *Fabio* does. In this way, you don't break contact with the G-Spot, but just alter it a bit. You basically continue the constant action within 'Me'arat HaMachpela,' but instead of a half-circle movement with your fingers (the 'come here' motion) inside *Angelina's* ceiling (the upper part of her vagina), they will now be doing the forward-backward motion in a straight line.

Remember

When you withdraw your fingers from deep inside the cave, there is no need to take them out completely or get to the exit itself. That way you're likely to miss the G-Spot and your woman will 'lose height.' (And your hand doesn't really need that right now, does it?) The goal is to move your fingers in and out with a very short range of motion and give *Angelina* the continuity she needs to get to the well and also drink from it…

A tip to conclude:

You can and should simultaneously combine the two methods – 'Me'arat HaMachpela' and 'Rosh HaNikra' – to achieve ultimate pleasure.

This does require highly developed coordination, but not on the level of a circus tightrope walker.

After all, if you succeeded at fulfilling the task of identifying the 'Miracle Button' and G-Spot, the rest is no big deal. So, go on, get to work, and remember: What doesn't walk on foot, goes on its hands – so give your fingers the chance to 'walk' in your place. Have a nice trip...

'The Rubbing Song'

The work to pleasure *Fabio* is much simpler and easier than that of pleasuring *Angelina*. Maybe this is due to the fact that *Angelina* is the daughter of Norwegian royalty, and men are less busy with 'royal poses,' or maybe it's just that *Fabio* is a large, easily located external limb, whereas *Angelina* is tiny and concealed by 'stalagmites' and devoted, ever-ready 'security guards.'

Practice only when wet:

A well-known subject in physics is the 'Friction Coefficient' – the less friction that exists between two bodies, the easier, faster and smoother the movement between them will be.

The same principle applies to sex: When you rub your hands, intending to provide *Fabio* with full and all-inclusive treatment, take into account that if your hand is not lubricated enough, he is likely to suffer instead of enjoying the touch of your beloved hand.

The human hand is indeed equipped with a natural lubrication system – a type of oil (not sweat) that is secreted onto the skin for the purpose of minimizing friction, but – unfortunately – it's not enough for the task at-hand.

Therefore, if you want to delight your *Rabbit*, and not abuse him or his *Fabio*, we recommend that you wet the 'naughty rod' with your saliva before giving the treatment. You can help your hand, using your mouth or tongue, as long as you make sure to be completely alert and aware that *Fabio* receives the necessary moisture throughout the entire deed. In other words, after you've lubricated him effectively, continue to pleasure him, but make sure to water him a second time, a moment before the liquid is absorbed and he is about to dry up again. Another way to moisturize the 'protruding rod' is to use body lotion or face cream (preferred). Face cream is certainly an expensive product, but we recommend you give *Fabio* the ten thousand dollar treatment as long as he's still 'riding,' otherwise he's likely to dry up or suffer from skin spots on his sensitive skin-wrapping. An additional advantage to the body lotion/face cream is that it is likely to lubricate *Fabio* through the entire job; you'll only need to arrange a 're-lubrication' in rare cases. Just between us, as long as you've already begun 'indulging the carrot,' an enthusiastic *Rabbit* won't feel any difference between body lotion, face cream or any other lubricant, but you will. And as a *Rabbit* who's suffered from drying out, I recommend avoiding mishaps along the way. 'Smooth out' the trip up through to the very top of the exploding volcano...

The Silk Road

Another important detail is tenderness of the touch. *Fabio* is indeed a mischievous creature, but he is actually the most sensitive of *Rabbit's* organs. Therefore, it's important that your touch be especially gentle, **and under no condition can you use your nails!!!**

Nails are certainly an attractive and sexy thing, but putting them into *Fabio* can make him shrivel up in size, hurt him, or even injure him, and the outcome will be ruining a wonderful evening, and maybe even chasing *Fabio* back into his tunnel for a very long time... you hear me *Jessica*?

A few moments of kindness

Before you 'get to it,' there is another small detail that should be dealt with – the male ego. Every *Rabbit* is happy to know how much you love his carrot, and the sooner he knows it, the better.

This is a very natural thing. Everyone needs to feel loved, even

Fabio, who looks totally 'full of himself'...

Therefore, if you want to calm your partner down before 'shifting' his gear stick, prove what a big fan you are of 'Mister Carrot' and show him how 'Roger Rabbit' gets trippy.

You probably already know how it is... every *Rabbit* wants to know that his carrot is the longest, the widest, and the best looking. And those that love *Fabio* get loved back many times over. So, the real question is, why not?

All you have to do is begin with light and gentle caresses, with your fingers half touching and half hovering. Stroke *Fabio* lovingly. Stimulate him and his beloved testicles, massage them slowly, and carefully caress the area between the testicles and the anus (also known as the scrotum; it's a particularly sensitive area). Continue spoiling him with every extravagant pleasure your hand comes up with...

Did you know?

Tickling *Fabio*, the testicles or the scrotum (the area between the testicles and the anus) while giving a hand-job can exponentially increase the *Rabbit's* pleasure. By doing this, you can easily become a Major in the field of 'indulgence' for the army's 'southern' division.

The Secret Foursome

There is an unlimited number of ways to pleasure your man. *Fabio* is a flexible and friendly character, and I'm sure he'll happily accept any technique you come up with – as long as you make sure he's safe and protected.

It doesn't really matter to *Rabbit* how you pamper his carrot, as long as you lubricate him, keep your sharp fingernails away and return him to his owner in exactly the same condition that you got him in.

There are a few leading and preferred techniques for treating the common carrot. And that's why your caring sisters have rolled up their sleeves and gathered four particularly effective and pleasure-filled techniques, so that you won't hit unnecessary embarrassment when you go face-to-face with the protruding, curious *Fabio*.

It all starts with positioning

First of all, you should begin your 'Rubbing Song' when you and your *Rabbit* are calm and relaxed.

A comfortable, liberated sitting position is an important detail for the upcoming 'opera', and the recommended position is to sit next to your partner, just below his butt, and facing him. Another suggested position is to sit between the *Rabbit's* open legs, facing him, and if you can, spread your legs a little so that the excited little guy can look at your shy *Angelina*. This will certainly begin the 'opera' with extraordinarily high pitches.

And now, the four techniques that will paint a thick, serene smile on his face:

Finger on the Trigger

Using this method (which is the most highly recommended and intense of them!), the hand-job is performed by you grabbing the lower section of *Fabio's* base with your lubricated hands – meaning, four fingers hold onto *Fabio's* lower segment from the side between *Fabio* and *Rabbit's* stomach. Put your thumb, which remains free, up against *Fabio's* other side at a 90 degree angle (this is the side between *Fabio* and your stomach) – meaning, you've created roughly a straight line from the tip of your thumb and the glans. Now you can begin!

Move your hand up along the length of the excited 'gear stick', stop the hand movement when your thumb is about two millimeters away from the head of the penis and continue with just your thumb.

Using your thumb, make a clockwise circle if you are working with your right hand, and move counterclockwise if you are using your left hand.

Return the thumb to its original spot in the exact same manner, and just like before, go straight down and then immediately move up again. Now, your thumb is back in its place about two millimeters below the head and closes its grip around *Fabio*.

After you've united your thumb with the other fingers, do the retreat motion and go down again to *Fabio's* lower section. At this stage, your fingers which are grasping the carrot move down toward its trunk (without touching the balls!). From that point, begin the entire process again…

This technique, which is consistently gaining more fans around the world, is capable of turning an apathetic *Rabbit* into a happy, satisfied creature. While it certainly isn't simple to do in the beginning, it also doesn't need a particularly high level of coordination. The second you internalize the finger movement, it becomes easier to do.

Remember

Don't loosen your grip on *Fabio* at any stage of the 'Rubbing Work.' That interferes with *Rabbit's* enjoyment. To allow *Fabio* to enjoy himself throughout the pampering, continue using a constant, uninterrupted action until the 'volcano explodes'…

The Gifted Class

For advanced students who have become adept at this technique and are interested in having *Rabbit* come faster, we recommend working just on *Fabio's* head and not the entire 'stick.' Meaning, the thumb motion and the other fingers focus on *Fabio's* upper area and do not handle the carrot's base. This promises your hypnotized *Rabbit* quick satisfaction with incredible pleasure. However, you should be aware that some men have trouble with this method due to 'over enjoyment' which is also likely to irritate them. Therefore, we suggest asking your *Rabbit* which method he prefers.

Power of the Buttonhole

The grip is not supposed to be gentle, but felt properly; still, make sure it isn't too strong. The idea is to give *Fabio* a treat and make him feel like he's in good hands, without causing a loss of blood supply. It's a well-known fact that there's a direct connection between the force of the grasp and *Fabio's* reaction time on his way to peaking. Still, you need a degree of sensitivity – try to identify the border between what will delight and speed up *Rabbit's* orgasm and what will hurt, aggravate and shrivel your *Fabio*. In other words, 'Pull the Carrot!' but only so much...

The trance tempo

The idea is to start at a slow and easygoing rhythm, and gradually increase it, so that at the end you are working so fast that your *Rabbit* goes into a trance. If you want your partner to fly so high he reaches the sky, keep a slow, relaxed pace with an average speed – not too fast but not too slow; the *Rabbit's* release will sound like a meteor crash. Unfortunately, however, most men aren't endowed with the attribute called patience. Therefore, if your *Rabbit* also suffers from this syndrome, continue increasing the speed until you launch him into outer-space with a big, satisfied smile. Now go on, get to work!

Reaction speed

An additional point that also must be considered is if *Fabio* reacts too quickly. The faster and stronger your handiwork, the faster *Fabio* will get to his anticipated release. A strong grip is likely to speed up *Rabbit's* orgasm, but you shouldn't bring it on too quickly. *Rabbits* are very sensitive about premature ejaculation. It hurts their self-image and that of their 'Wonder Carrot.' And we wouldn't want to have a frightened *Rabbit*. So, you should always make sure to balance between the desire to have your partner enjoy and climax, and rushing him to come when *Rabbit* hasn't yet had enough time to enjoy.

One hand washes the other

To do this terrific technique, start by oiling up both of your hands, as well as *Fabio,* the recipient of this treat. Doing this will ensure your partner a juicy celebration.

With one hand, grab *Fabio's* upper end and begin moving downward, until you've almost arrived at his testicles. When you are close to the mischievous pair, release your hand grip (before you touch the testicles), grab the top of *Fabio* with your second hand, move downward, and repeat. It is very important that your hands work simultaneously and don't leave *Fabio* alone for more than half a second. In other words: when your first hand reaches *Fabio's* base, the second hand quickly grabs the top and does exactly the same motion as the hand before it, and so on and so forth. To avoid causing *Fabio* any pain, you must always do the same 'gliding movement' downward and not switch directions.

Continue to work in this way with one hand going down from the top of the carrot, stopping at the balls, and the second hand continuing with the exact the same action. Your partner will convulse with pleasure. Trust me.

Using power, not brainpower

As everything is related to the grip strength, you can forcefully tighten your hands around the upper end of the oily 'rod.' Of course, you should use some level of care. The purpose is to give *Fabio* a good time, not to turn him into a wet blanket.

Let's hear some music

In this method, much like the previous technique, we recommend starting with a slow pace, 'to get into the game' and then continue increasing the speed until the explosive finale. Of course, as far as *Rabbit* is concerned, a slow, sensual effort is preferred; it increases the intensity when he comes. But, as I already emphasized earlier, most *Rabbits* aren't very patient when it comes to a 'challenged' carrot, and so, if you see that your partner is already heading toward the light at the end of the tunnel, go with his flow.

Exposed inside the Castle

Here again, start off your indulgent deed with two well-lubricated hands.

Intertwine the fingers of your hands so that the bottoms of your palms are up against one another and your intertwined fingers create a small space meant for dear *Fabio*. Position your hands on *Fabio's* upper end, place him between your fingers and, in the special gap you've created, begin moving your intertwined hands down to the carrot stem without touching the balls. When you've arrived at your destination, go back up and repeat the action over and over again until the sweet Happy Ending.

A time to squeeze and a time to loosen up

The power of the grip changes from section to section when using this interesting technique. While gliding downward, as your hands close in on *Fabio* from the head down the shaft (the lowest section), squeeze hard. However, when you move up, and get to the lower section of the glans (the foreskin area), ease the pressure to a light hold, so that you won't hurt poor *Rabbit*. From here on, you can move back down and again increase the pressure, with the goal of increasing your partner's enjoyment.

Not too difficult, right? Ask *Rabbit* if he is able to talk after…

Divide and Conquer

The last, very likeable and slightly adventurous technique will leave devoted *Fabio* in one hand and the sociable testicles in your other. And now, to the jerking operation!

Lubricate both your hands well (so as to not hurt *Fabio* or accidentally tear a few rebellious hairs from his testicle area) and place one hand on each of the precious treasures. Grab *Fabio* lovingly with one hand and move it up and down – from the glans area to the praiseworthy shaft, and repeat.

With your second hand, gently grab the two testicles and gently, pull them outward. Do this as if (but only as if) you were trying to remove them from the body. Since this is a particularly sensitive body part for men, it is very important to make sure that your touch is extra gentle and that you avoid exerting hard pressure that will likely deactivate them for a while.

This action pulls *Fabio's* skin and increases the pleasure of your confused *Rabbit,* who will certainly not understand what the hell you are doing – but don't worry, he'll understand soon…

Another option that combines touching both *Fabio* and the balls involves raising the testicles (very gently) toward the carrot while indulging *Fabio* with your other hand.

You can be sure that your *Rabbit* will thank you for your interest in his two round pearls, and very quickly, you'll discover that the carrot is also very thankful – in his own liquid style.

Did you know?

Pressing on the scrotum – the area between the testicles and the anus (but closer to the testicles) – makes *Fabio* hard and erect. It also intensifies the *Rabbit's* pleasure, making him quickly water you with his love liquid.

A fun trick for you to try at home: Press on the area mentioned above and watch the hard banana jump for joy the second you take your finger off the spot.

Chapter 3

The King's Pool: Oral sex

Each of us loves feeling like someone wants us enough to be compelled to bend over and taste 'our love fruit' at-length. Aside from the heavenly enjoyment that comes from licking a sexual organ, it also offers a clear, unmistakable statement about how sexy and desirable we are.

So, diving down to the 'bottom of our pool' crowns us 'King' for one day and turns the sexual deed into an exciting and exhilarating one.

Almost everyone will be happy if their partner 'dives down to the bottom,' and there are those that even prefer this over the routine intercourse that brings *Fabio* and *Angelina* together. However, it's important to understand that good sex includes oral pleasure for both sides. If you are interested in being flawless lovers, we highly recommended that you learn the 'bottom of your partner's pool' well. This will definitely bring you closer together and will incomparably improve your sex.

For the 'first dip' into the pool, we recommend that you, Kings and Queens, return to the Chapter 'Clearing the Air' to refresh yourselves, renew your strengths and return to battle with a 'clear head.'

Licking the Toffee

One of the most exciting presents you can give a woman is to lick her 'toffee.' To hold the soft, pink candy in your mouth and suck it gently. Your Queen will feel loved, desirable and sexy. And if she has trouble climaxing in the conventional way, rest assured that licking her 'toffee' will do miracles. She will not only come with trumpets blaring, but will also beg for more every time you're alone.

Therefore, men, even if licking the 'toffee' isn't exactly your 'thing,' it's definitely worth your while to make it one. Your partners will enjoy themselves like you wouldn't believe, and will be ready to tell anyone willing to listen about the big lottery ticket they just won.

It's not too bad to be someone's winning ticket; is it? And especially if that someone is a Queen.

A few enchanted words before the magic begins

More than a few women are likely to feel uncomfortable about their bodies. They may be breath-taking princesses or Siamese cats dripping with sex appeal, and still feel that the King won't love their body, skin color, or smell. Because of this, they sometimes avoid giving access to their Norwegian princess, worrying that *Angelina* isn't pretty enough, doesn't smell as she should, or is perhaps 'flooded.'

Therefore, in order to 'connect' one on one with *Angelina*, we recommend complimenting the Queen on her impressive body and 'going down' to the details about her different body parts: their shape, their color, their smell and everything, of course, is said just the right amount. We wouldn't want to exaggerate and make the Queen think our words are worth as little as garlic peel.

The correct amount of compliments will soften the 'mistress' up, boost her self-confidence and help her open the gates that lead into *Angelina's* bedroom.

'Flow Chart'

To help you 'float' easily in the King's Pool, I now refer you to the Chapter 'Nice Rubbing' for a short, but effective, description of *Angelina's* structure.

Preparing the terrain

Before giving our undivided attention to *Angelina*, the peripheral areas should also be well taken care of. Progressing slowly is very important – the slower you dive down toward the bottom, the more your Queen will enjoy herself. Expectation is a wonderful thing, and in sex, even more so. We recommend going progressively further down her body with your tongue toward the belly button; kiss, bite lightly, and lovingly lick everything on the way including the stomach, hip bones, thighs, and skin next to the crotch. At this point, you are welcome to gently blow on the areas that you wet with your tongue. This feels cool and nice as it chills the body.

After you wet most of the southern area, continue on the 'King's path' – the area between *Angelina* and the anus. Only after you've finished fully exciting your Queen are you invited to briefly visit the Norwegian princess herself. Once again, to add excitement we recommend that you 'visit but don't arrive;' however, from the second you've made full contact with *Katie*, you should continue without letting her rest so that she won't 'dry up' and lose interest.

Landing on Mars

After you've landed on the 'Miracle Button,' Mars feels hotter and hotter with excitement, look at it, be impressed by the incredibly feminine design, and begin to gently stroke every part of *Angelina* with your fingertips.

Next, begin working with your mouth: Before you get to the 'Miracle Button' – the clitoris, you should begin by 'warming up' in the whole area. Lick the outer labia, the inner labia and the 'Me'arat HaMachpela' – the hole at the back end *Angelina*. Let me tell you – Queens go into total ecstasy when you put your tongue into the 'Me'arat HaMachpela.' It blinds them with pleasure. Move your tongue in and out a few times, or at the very least twice each time, and continue to lick the area slowly and sensually. Your Queen will appreciate it.

Slow is the name of the game. This way you show your partner that you're enjoying yourself no less than she is. And, that your entire body is burning with desire for her and her *Angelina*. Kiss, lick, nibble, caress and penetrate your fingers into *Katie*, just like you learned to do in 'Nice Rubbing.'

The Cherry on Top

After having a few minutes of romance with *Angelina* and her 'periphery,' the time has come to shift gears and set a date with the 'Miracle Button' – the main course for pleasuring a woman. It's important to note that for most women, the 'Miracle Button' is very sensitive. And therefore, it's best that you don't lift up the skin covering it, but instead thrill the 'Button' along with its crown.

However, there are some women who do prefer contact on their exposed clitoris. In these cases, you should lift the clitoral glans – using your upper lip – toward the Queen's breasts and expose the clitoris. If your partner loves direct contact, she will quiver with joy when your tongue licks her 'Button' without any middle men. In either case, communication between you two is invaluably important. You should ask the Queen about her preferences, making her feel that her prince is interested in her and her desires, and that he is ready to do anything to improve the 'summit.'

At the beginning, you can put your tongue up against the clitoris. Make it relaxed and not pursed, and leave it there without moving for a few seconds. This way you can relax your partner and prepare her for the 'tongue acrobatics' that are about to come.

Climbing onto the trapeze

And now, for the 'Main Show:'

There are many different methods for doing 'acrobatics' on the 'Miracle Button':

- **The Pendulum Effect**: Place the edge of your tongue on

the clitoris and move it right and left, over and over again.

- **The Elevator Affect**: Place the edge of your tongue on the clitoris and move it back and forth, again and again. It's important to note that this method is a bit harder than the last one for the tongue muscles. But because it is very indulgent and makes her feel dizzy, it's definitely worthwhile.

Tempo

With both methods, start slow and progressively increase the speed. Reach your maximum speed at the end.

Force

Here as well, we recommend beginning with a relatively weak motion and increasing progressively. Make sure you constantly pay attention to the Queen's reactions. If she doesn't seem to be calm, lower the pressure, since the goal is to pleasure her and not cause her pain.

'O mama': Put your lips around the 'Miracle Button' in an 'O' shape and vacuum her mildly in your mouth. You should suck, release for a hundredth of a second to take air, and then return again to your delicious 'toffee.'

If your partner shows signs of increasing pleasure, you should increase the power of the 'suckling' until you've reached her desired level.

Love bites: Another method is to gently bite (very gently!) the clitoris with small, occasional bites as you're doing licking. This won't make the Queen come, but it will definitely help her to get there.

As noted earlier, every woman likes for you to 'dive into her pool' differently. One Queen will prefer the 'Pendulum Affect,' another likes the 'Elevator Affect,' a third the 'O Mama' and a fourth sucking and licking together. From here on in, it's your job to test your partner's preferences according to her body's reactions, and to match the technique, tempo and force to her.

Our recommendation: Begin by using the Pendulum or Elevator Effect for up to a minute, move on to the 'O Mama' for a small amount of time and then go back and continue until the end using either the first or second technique – depending on what the Queen prefers.

Most important

When your Queen has already entered her ecstasy, under no circumstances can you change the technique, pace or force. You must continue exactly as you are until she reaches the heavenly orgasm awaiting her.

Some Queens will finish quickly, while others come slowly. Everything happens according to their biological structure, and level of comfort with their body. Don't speed her up – it will come on its own…

Acrobatics

At this point, we've collected three terrific positions that will bump you up from average 'Olympic swimmers' to proud medal owners. There are, of course, other positions and you can let your imaginations go crazy. But, you should know the 'divas' of this domain well:

- **An Eye for an Eye**: This is the most comfortable position. The Queen lies on her back with her legs spread, and you kneel between her legs facing her. To make the position even better, you can rest a pillow under the Queen's hips, thereby lifting the entire area and giving you easier access to *Angelina*.
- **Sixty-nine**: This wonderful position is done when one of the partners lies on their back, and the other lies on top, reversed. The stomachs touch one another, but the face of each partner is in front of the other's genitals. In other

words: The man's face is looking directly at *Angelina,* and the woman's face is near *Fabio.* This is a wonderful position because both *Fabio* and *Angelina* benefit from simultaneous, shared team work done by the King and Queen.

If you're interested in stimulating the Queen's G-spot while licking her 'toffee,' then this position is not recommended for you. Either way, we recommend that you go back and reread 'Nice Rubbing,' to update yourself with effective techniques we've suggested for that purpose.

- **The T**: For this position, the Queen lies on her back, legs spread with a pillow resting under her hips. You come in from the side and rest your head above *Angelina*. (If we were to compare the situation to the letter T, you are essentially the leg). You can lick the 'toffee' exactly like in the Pendulum Effect, but the Queen will feel as if you're doing the Elevator Effect.

Trouble on the road to heaven:

Rest for the Weary: The process of coming is slow for some women, and so, positions 1 and 2 are likely to tire out your tongue muscles. However, you are absolutely prohibited from stopping before the Queen has climaxed, since this will quickly plummet her back down to the ground from the heavenly heights your generous tongue has flown her to. Therefore, at this stage of 'material fatigue,' you can do the 'O Mama' effect and suck your partner's clitoris for a little while. This will give your tongue a break and muster up energy so you can return to the holy work.

Another trick 'for a tongue vacation' is stretching the tongue out of the mouth as far as it can go. It must be pointed downward, toward your chin, and rest there. Now, you continue to work using the neck muscles instead of the tongue muscles. Move your head up and down over the Queen's 'Miracle Button' so that your tongue brushes against *Angelina* between her outer labia (through to the clitoris).

An alternative based on the previous trick again involves sticking your tongue out and using the neck muscles instead of the tongue. The novelty here is that when the tongue is at *Angelina's* lower section in 'Me'arat HaMachpela,' it stretches out as far as it can go; when the head moves up in front of the 'Rosh HaNikra' area, the tongue retracts almost completely into the mouth. This increases the friction with *Angelina* and also gives you the benefit of another second of rest at the end of the process. Keep in mind that the tongue has to touch the 'Miracle Button' every time it passes, and only afterwards returns to the anus area.

With time, the more you practice and acquire experience, the stronger and more-skilled your tongue will become. Sooner or later you won't need the tricks anymore. You'll be able to get your partner to climax in one continuous, non-stop act.

Political asylum: Toward the end, you are likely to feel the 'Miracle Button' run away and disappear in the midst of the action. Don't worry! It isn't running to ask *Angelina* for political asylum. This is a completely natural, biological process that stems from the clitoris' extreme sensitivity, and it indicates that your partner is about to 'reach the stars.' We highly recommend that you continue with exactly the same technique and direction that you're using, so that your Queen experiences an exceptional orgasm.

Whoever starts has to finish: Even though we've already said this before, it's important to give this issue a paragraph of its own so that you can internalize it completely. Never under any condition can you stop in the middle of the oral pleasure-giving, even if your Queen begins to 'gather mileage' before the end. This will ruin everything and bring her level of stimulation down to the ground. And why? All you have to do is continue using the exact same position. Meaning: If you're in the process of one tongue motion, continue using it until the bitter end. You can increase the pace or the intensity (within reason – using too much force will ruin the pleasure), which will help the Queen to cross the finish line successfully.

You can't argue over taste or smell: If *Angelina's* flavor or smell is not tasty to your palate or nice on your nose, return to the chapter on 'Clearing the Air' and read it over again. As an additional step, you can bring your Queen into the shower and 'clear the air' during an intimate pampering session. Wash intimate or regular soap across *Angelina*, soap up the Norwegian princess, lather up the 'Miracle Button' gently, wash the area with water and fly back to the bed.

Rule of the Intertwined Vessels:

As you probably already know, working simultaneously with the tongue and fingers is very important. This is connected to the fact that every woman has a different preference. There are those that come only when gone down upon, others from fingering or penetration, and the majority from a synchronized combination of the two. So, if you want to make sure that you successfully please your Queen, and also as a 'shortcut,' we recommend that on first contact with a partner you use a few different methods. Before describing the stages of execution, I suggest you use both hands simultaneously. If that's not possible, one hand is certainly enough.

The stages to do on your path to pleasuring the bottom of 'King's Pool' with your tongue are:

Start by having one hand wander slowly across the length of the Queen's body, gently caressing her face, stomach and chest. Move a finger across her face and put it into her mouth. Sucking the finger will wake your partner up, as it will remind her (and you) of dear *Fabio*.

At this point, your other hand (either simultaneously or afterward) pleasures *Angelina* (according to what you learned in 'Nice Rubbing'). While your hand is pleasuring *Angelina*, it's very important that it works directly on the G-Spot, as this is the critical stage in the 'dive.' The combination of fingering and skilled craftsmanship with the tongue will lead to an incredible, unprecedented orgasm.

Throughout the dive, we recommend that you try and penetrate your finger into the Queen's 'kitchenette' – the anus. It's best for you to check and see how she reacts to this, instead of surprising her with a quick, sharp movement. Many women love it, but there are those that have never tried 'back penetration' and so, don't know if they are for or against. Either way, as you'll learn in the 'Kitchenette,' when your Queen's *Angelina* region is 'well oiled,' the moisture also trickles back to the 'kitchenette' area. This makes finger penetration into the anus much easier.

Epilogue

If you're interested in being the ideal lover, there are a few things we recommend you do after the big sex flames subside a bit:

When the Queen's body language indicates that she has climaxed, or alternatively, if she pushes your head away from her *Angelina* with her hands, it's best not to move or make any sudden movements. If your fingers are deep within the 'Me'arat HaMachpela,' leave them there for a bit (at least a minute) and allow your partner to rest, relax and come back to her senses.

After your Queen has calmed down, move up, lie next to her and give her a soft, loving hug, along with a gentle kiss on the mouth.

Now, after you've shown your Queen how much you love her, this is the time to go down and show her the love once again. Go back and delight *Angelina* with your tongue, sending her into a second, wonderful and no less dizzying orgasm.

Many women, as opposed to men, are able to experience multiple orgasms consecutively. Some of them enjoy if you go down on them a second time immediately after the first orgasm, but most prefer that you wait a few minutes and allow *Angelina* to collect herself before the upcoming 'storm.'

There are women that will greatly enjoy alternately penetrating *Angelina* and licking the 'toffee.' This is an especially great mix, especially if you studied the 'Just a bit before we finish…' about how to come after your Queen.

We recommend that you 'shift gears' relatively quickly between going down on her and penetration, so that you don't lose momentum and calm the Queen down. However, we do of course recommend that you don't do it too fast so that you don't hurt your partner during the transition between the two positions.

Diving Forward

Men, just like women, need a shot of encouragement along with the feeling that they are sexy, desirable and loved. One of the ways to make your King understand just how much you're attracted to him and his 'athletic friend' is by using oral sex – or, 'diving down to the bottom of his pool.'

We wholeheartedly recommend that you dedicate some of the sex to oral activity. This increases the intensity of sex between you and your King, and also makes him feel like your undisputed 'Elvis.'

Men, as understood by the rule of nature, will always come; even if the treatment their *Fabio* received wasn't perfect or fantastic. However, a large percentage of men all over the world do complain that women aren't well-informed enough about 'diving' work. Therefore, ladies, if you want to be unique, and prove to your Kings that that's one big piece of bullshit, then you should treat this chapter seriously and internalize it. Following your partner's professional 'licking the horse,' he'll feel like he switched an antique jalopy for a new Mercedes.

It's important to explain that learning the three techniques in this chapter thoroughly takes patience.

For this reason, excited Kings hold your horses and give your partners some time and leeway.

The journey itself is just as important as the destination

During the 'dive down to your King's bottom,' it's important for you to take your time and not hurry. Don't get to the main part – 'licking the horse' – immediately; instead, procrastinate first with the view along the way… and drive your King crazy. Let him suck on your finger, make your tongue wander across the length of his stomach, come close to 'Fabio,' continue on to the leg, nibble, kiss, lick, caress, blow some cool air on the wet areas, and do everything you can think of to make your partner lose his mind with pleasure.

We recommend licking or tickling the testicles (but never biting them!!!), continuing with your tongue or fingers to the 'kitchenette' (anus), and by doing this, increasing and arousing your King's appetite for the 'main course.'

If you want to calm your partner down and let him know that you plan on diving down toward his *Fabio* during sex (an important and significant subject among the Kings), you can always start with a kiss or nice lick on *Fabio* and from there on, continue with your game in being impressed by the 'beautiful views' along the way.

That being said, from the moment you get to dear *Fabio* and begin the 'tongue action,' you should stay there and not continue onward so that our *Fabio* won't cool off and lose his urge.

Show him what a 'professional diver' you are that you won't stop until the King's 'love fluids' have filled the pool.

From the instructors all the way to the finish line

Since *Fabio* isn't endowed with *Angelina's* 'automatic self-lubrication,' you should wet him throughout the 'dive.' You can do this easily with a large amount of saliva which will completely eliminate any problematic friction.

Carnal lust

Every woman that intends to orally pleasure her King should forget about her teeth and begin with 'carnal lust' – contact between *Fabio* and her lips alone. Touching your teeth to the King's 'horse' can destroy his enjoyment completely and ruin the sensual atmosphere that you've moved into. So, you cannot bite *Fabio* or involve your teeth in the 'diving down to the bottom' process.

For those of you that don't know the lip motion during the 'dive' stage and don't know how to do it without using your teeth, here's a small trick that will help your situation: Close your lips and make sure that your teeth don't touch each other. Now open your mouth gradually and leave it half-closed.

Now, all that's left for you to do is do this same action when you're planning to lick the King's *Fabio*, and you're totally covered.

Techniques for Treating the Snorkel

Before we send you, dear students, to 'dive' toward the bottom of the 'King's Pool,' we should first equip you with a few techniques for treating the snorkel – just to make sure that it's a good, satisfying dive. First of all, it's important to remember that one of the most significant subjects in the dive process is giving your partner the feeling that you enjoy 'licking the horse' and are in awe of the impressive, seductive thing hanging between his legs.

Here are three fantastic techniques that will turn your Kings into particularly smiley, satisfied men.

Going down to Mexico

This is the easiest way to give head. And, the orgasm your King experiences will be one of the best he's ever had.

The pleasure of going slow: It's very important to do the 'dive' at an indulgently slow pace, licking *Fabio* patiently. This will definitely pay off during the King's over-the-top finish. Like we said earlier, the journey is just as important as the destination. And, so, take your time and allow your woman, dear King, to do her work in her slow, indulgent manner.

The Essence of the Essence: Now we're arrived at the essence, at the moment of truth – the stage at which you actually learn how to make the King's aroused 'snake' dance inside your mouth.

Before we begin, we'll let you women know that the Mexican method needs a lot of lubrication (saliva or any other oil) to minimize the friction that's problematic for *Fabio*.

And now the explanation: Tighten your lips gently around *Fabio*. Try to do this steadily, meaning not too lightly but also not too strong. Put your tongue up against it (but make sure that the tongue stays in your mouth and does not cross the line of your lips).

Now, with your lips and tongue in the desired location, move your head as far down as you can, come back up, and so on and so forth. In principle, *Fabio's* head is a very sensitive area, and so, we suggest that you go down halfway (to *Fabio's* middle) and then go back up again and pleasure the 'fox head.'

In addition to the calculated work done by the tongue and lips, there's a need for gentle, skilled handiwork. Tighten your hand gently (not too lightly but still delicately) around *Fabio* and move it up and down at the same time as your lips (either with them or in the opposite direction).

Once in a while, you can move your head right or left to create an angle that will increase *Fabio's* enjoyment. Additionally, know that the longer you go down on him, the stronger 'Elvis' will come. So, we recommend taking your time.

Since this method needs to be very gentle, it takes a relatively long time, but justifies every second. You should try to relax your King, who will certainly want his orgasm quickly. But, in the long term, he'll greatly appreciate it.

For men whose orgasms tend to take a while, are impatient or are simply further along in the race compared to the rest of the pack – you can combine this with the 'Finger on the Trigger' method found in the chapter called 'Nice Rubbing.' The moment your lips go up the length of *Fabio* and lift off from him, your thumb starts its role doing work on the 'fox head.' Immediately afterward, your lips return to *Fabio*, go down as far as possible, and repeat. It is most important to make sure *Fabio* isn't neglected for even a second. Make sure he is under the constant supervision of either your hand or lips.

To minimize the time before he comes, tighten your hand more around *Fabio*, but don't do it so much that you strangle the 'guest of honor.'

The Spiral Descent

In this technique, just like the previous one, wetting *Fabio* is very important since the contact between him and the hand and lips is very intensive.

The Essence of the Essence: The idea in Spiral Descent is that you can basically use 'Going down to Mexico' as your foundation, but your lips (and tongue) are tightened more firmly around *Fabio*, and the hand-job is done in a twisting-motion simultaneously. Here too your hand moves up and down over the length of *Fabio*, but in a twist rotation of ninety degrees – beginning from when your hand grabs his base and until it gets to his beautiful head. In other words, the twist-rotations are not done in place, but over the entire length. Also, the grip on *Fabio* is not meant to be strong, since the skin is stretched throughout the twist which could hurt the sensitive prince. For this very reason, dear ladies, when your hand goes down from *Fabio's* smooth head to his base, it should be done in a straight line and not with a twist.

Important note: The hand and head should be coordinated

while applying the spiral technique. When the head goes down, the hand should also go down; and when it goes up, the hand does too. However, women wanting to give oral pleasure just to *Fabio's* head are welcome to focus their mouth in sucking on the prince's head and doing the spiral hand-job with their hand. Additionally, there are men who prefer that you suck on *Fabio's* head instead of combining the twist motion with the 'Going down to Mexico.' The idea is for the hand to go down during the sucking, and for your mouth to rest when it moves up, but not leave *Fabio's* head.

Going down to Denmark/England

This time as well, the issue of timing is invaluably important. First, ladies, in order to become skilled in this interesting technique, you have to practice and acquire the ability and professionalism over time. Second, dear men, take into account that during her application of this technique, it will take you a few minutes to understand what your baby wants to do. Be patient, this will prove itself all the way to your wonderful orgasm.

It's possible that *Fabio* will be slightly irritated and may even hurt the next day, but this is definitely a trivial sacrifice to pay for the pure joy that the Descent to Denmark/England gives you.

Essence of the Essence:

a Tighten the thumb and index finger around *Fabio* strongly in the area under and near the foreskin (leave enough space for your lips which will suck on *Fabio's* head). The grip must be particularly strong. It should be a bit more than what you think is the very limit of your King's ability. Get rid of any doubt – you are not hurting him, just stopping the flow of blood to *Fabio's* smooth, beautiful head.

b Now, tighten your lips around *Fabio's* head and go down

the entire length, until you reach your fingers that are wrapped around it; but do not pass them. Tighten them powerfully around *Fabio* and suck him as hard as you do a lollipop. Suck him with power, release, suck and release again. Continue again and again without ever removing your lips from him (meaning the release is from the sucking and not of *Fabio*).

c After at least a minute, release your finger grip for fifteen seconds, and then, perfectly timed to the release of your grip, suck especially hard.

d Immediately after, hold your grip (exactly as described in Section A) for ten seconds and continue 'sucking the lollipop.'

e After ten seconds, repeat the exercise. In other words, release your grip, 'pump' Fabio with dual power, retighten your grip, continue 'sucking the lollipop' and repeat until he's reached the much-awaited climax.

We recommend placing a fluffy pillow under your King's head, since he will fling his head back every time you release your magical grip and do the infamous 'pumping.' If you don't have any pillows in the house, you should have band-aids ready since his head is going to get really banged up with the tempo reserved for Denmark/England.

It's important to note that not every King will get attached to this slightly aggressive technique. So, if your partner begins to complain, leave Europe and try to discover Mexico.

Acrobatics

I've gathered two basic, but effective positions for doing your Olympic work. They are simple, practical and exceptional.

As we've already said to your Kings, there are other positions and you can use your wild imagination to create any shape and style you see fit.

A leg here, a leg there: Your King lies on his back with open legs, and you lie between his legs, with your head facing his.

Sixty Nine: A wonderful and highly recommended position for both sides (See the section on 'Acrobatics' for women earlier in this chapter).

And to conclude the chapter: The very last drops

Dear sisters! You should know that Kings are different from one another. There are those that love when you 'Go Down to Mexico,' others prefer 'Going to Denmark/England,' and some love them both. From here on in, a part of your work is trial and error – until you either hit the target or use the easiest and more direct approach of asking your partner what he prefers.

If your King is dawdling and his orgasm is slow in coming, constant pressure of intermediate force on the pipe swollen between the testicles and the anus will take him to the 'holy land' much quicker than you think.

We recommend not licking *Fabio's* slippery head for too long, and in principle, not focusing on the same spot either, since this pleasures him at the start, but becomes an irritation the longer it continues.

If you want your King's orgasm to be wonderful and unprecedented, keep him from coming!

How?

A few seconds before his orgasm comes, stop the oral and hand work. Wait thirty seconds and continue until 'almost' the next one... repeat this a few times (with the assumption that your King is patient enough) and get ready for a mega-orgasm – a crazy, enormous nuclear explosion. Of course, it's important to know your partner. If you stop half a second after his 'no return' point (see 'A second before we finish') you're likely to irreparably sabotage his orgasm.

Important note

This suggestion is irrelevant when you are 'Going Down to Mexico,' since your King has waited long enough and he doesn't have time for unnecessary delays.

Dear Sisters: An important part of pleasuring your Kings is watching the operations you've plotted. So, for those of you with long hair, pull it back while you are 'licking the hose' and give your fiery King some added excitement and desire.

Slip of the tongue

As you know, there are claims for and against ejaculating the Sultan's sperm by his partner.

Men claim that it's important to them to climax in their partner's mouth, since it gives them great pleasure and doesn't ruin their orgasm, and a large portion of women, are opposed to swallowing the sperm as they don't love the taste.

We've collected for you, gorgeous Kings and Queens, two claims for swallowing sperm, an alternative solution, in the case that we're talking about a particularly stubborn Sultana, and a few methods for improving the taste of the sperm: Studies claim that the man's sperm has ingredients in it that help prevent depression in women. The Sunday Times published a study that claims swallowing male sperm regularly improves concentration by 34 percent, is effective for skin, burns calories and lessens tension due to the high concentration of minerals found in sperm.

When your partner finishes 'licking the hose' a second before the orgasm and continues with a handjob, the King's enjoyment is significantly smaller:

First, until she continues with the handjob, momentum is lost and the strength of the orgasm has decreased. Second, even if the King is at his 'no return' point, he will come much more weakly than he could have.

The Solution

It is important to clarify that this is not a perfect solution, but in any case, it is better than nothing.

All that you have to do is grab Fabio firmly with your hand, and go up and down the length with increasing speed a few seconds before you take your lips off of him. And so, after the separation, you continue the masturbation until the awaited orgasm. Your King will feel the difference between the oral indulgence and hand pampering, but this method will ensure a desirable and strong climax for him. It is important to note that the grip on Fabio must be continuous and consecutive. A break, no matter how short, will return him to the start point. You've been warned!

Methods for improving the 'Love Fluid's' taste

Dear King, the smell and taste of your sperm are affected by your nutrition. So, healthy and organized meals that include: meat, fish, eggs and vegetables will improve the taste of your love fluid, and will mix better on your Queen's palate.

The more water you drink, the more the taste, smell and texture of your sperm will improve.

From here, both on days with heatwave and heavy rain, we recommend that you swallow plenty of water, even if you haven't been thirsty for a while.

Eating fruits, which are an aphrodisiac by themselves, will sweeten your 'cum' and will improve its taste without recognition. Coffee, however, will result in a bitter and troubled face from them, and this is not what you want in order to convince her that this is the 'Nectar of the Gods' that you're supplying.

Chapter 4

The Kitchenette

The 'Back Kitchenette,' better known as the anus (on both men and women) – is an area explored much less during sex in comparison to other parts of our bodies. And what a shame. Travelers who flinch at the idea of touring around this spot because of security concerns (thick fog clouds, sudden rainstorms, muddy ground, etc.) aren't aware of the many advantages offered in this wonderful 'valley' surrounded by two calm mountains. It is for those people that we now reiterate things said earlier to remind them of this book's motto: 'Don't be shy, just try!'

Given the overall population's minimal experience in anal activity, the explanations provided in this chapter will be more detailed and basic than others. It's important to note that the descriptions are directed both at women – for whom the act of anal sex can greatly enrich their sex lives, and at men – whose famous G-spot is located deep inside the 'kitchenette.' (Details can be found later on in this chapter).

Anal Sex

First we should note that anal sex isn't for everyone. If you love the missionary position, and prefer a calm cup of tea, then mix carefully and be well…

This chapter is recommended for those in search of stimulation and change, for those who prefer a well-blended orgasm, and, basically, to anyone interested in adding a new, exciting ingredient into their sex lives!

So – if you are sick of the banal, try the anal!

Did you know?

Why is it so enjoyable? A very high number of nerve endings are concentrated in the anus. Because of this, the spot is very sensitive to touch and, therefore, pleasure-filled and a place that affords a powerful, dizzying sexual experience.

A rule familiar to every new chef is the need to maintain a high-level of cleanliness before entering the kitchenette. Therefore, with the purpose of having a 'clean, smooth' entrance, we recommend you hold hands and once again browse through the Chapter called 'Clearing the Air.'

Instructions for Preparation

A tour around the 'kitchenette' is slow and gradual, as this is particularly mountainous and slippery terrain. Therefore, muster up your utmost amount of patience and perform each stage one at a time. Complete one stage for every session of sexual intercourse. (Keep in mind the Suez Canal wasn't dug in one day…).

The goal of the following stages is to turn the act of anal sex into a more pleasant and pleasure-filled one. Also, to expand the anus muscle so that later on, when it is more flexible and experienced, it will be prepared to let our mischievous friend *Fabio* come for a visit...

So, fasten your safety belts, put your hands together and walk around the kitchenette's mysterious crevices! It'll definitely be worth your while. The 'cherry on top' will be waiting at the end of your tour.

Stage One

The first stage and most important part of this process is relaxation. The act of anal sex is based on mutual trust and a complete sense of serenity. If your partner is not calm, the muscles of their anus will contract immediately; it will be impossible to penetrate anything into there, even a needle (and I really hope your ammunition amounts to more than that). For that reason, it's very important you don't go touring around everyone's 'kitchenette,' but instead only do this with a regular partner that you trust.

Stage Two or 'Long Tongue'

'The Lick,' otherwise known by its professional name as Rimming. 'The King's Path' (the area between the genitalia and the anus, all inclusive) is a very sensitive place that reacts wonderfully to touch (penetration or otherwise). We suggest licking it with every method you know – just as long as you do it softly and gently since this is the best way to act with a prince or princess.

Your partner will lose their senses when you lick their anal area, and most importantly: It will get them to relax and allow you to do anything you can think of to do while pleasuring them (see Stage One).

Bonuses for those delving into the material:

If you want to increase your partner's pleasure, rub the edge of your tongue over their anus again and again or penetrate your tongue as deep as possible inside. Then push it forward and back without separating from the anus throughout the entire act. Another way to stir up the 'kitchenette' is to rub your lips gently on the anus or to suck it forcefully. (Don't worry this will also wet other areas). This action is especially indulgent if combined with tongue penetration.

We also highly recommend combining the tongue concerto into the anal district with a 'massage' for your partner's genitals, so that they won't feel neglected or deprived. (This is what you learned in the Chapter 'Nice Rubbing.')

Kitchen owner: If while you receive the anal licking you do pushing motions (like when doing your 'solid' business, but only like… don't actually flood out onto your devoted partner's face). This will increase the outer area of your anus, providing an added slice for licking, nibbling, and delighting.

Stage Three or 'God's Fingers': The same delightful, tasty delicacies can also be cooked up with our loyal friend – the finger.

Very important

Since, as opposed to *Angelina*, the anal area is not naturally lubricated, you must wet your finger (or anything else that you penetrate into this sensitive region) with saliva, body oil or special body cream intended for penetration. We recommend not using materials that include soap out of concern that they may create an enema effect.

(Special oils can be purchased at sex shops, pharmacies, etc. Worst case scenario, you should use the oiliest cream you can find).

Play Maestro, play!

At first, penetrate using only one finger, preferably the pinkie – since it is the thinnest and smallest one.

You can do easy rotations during the penetration to warm up the 'engine,' but make sure that the penetration motion is done as gently and slowly as possible so that your partner will remain calm, relaxed and prepared for the 'gear shift.'

Throughout, be aware of how your partner reacts to the 'kitchen invasion.' If you sense discomfort or pain, stop immediately and put off continuing until another time. As we've already said in this chapter: patience pays off...

Congratulations! If you're at this stage, it means your finger has successfully penetrated.

Now, once you've penetrated your finger all the way to the end, you need to put it in and out repeatedly, just like in intercourse. Don't disconnect completely from the anus. (Be sure to leave a part of the finger inside at all times, much like conventional penetration into *Angelina*).

Important tip: Do not, under any circumstances, wear a ring on the penetrating finger. Also, make sure the nail on that finger isn't long (see 'Clearing the Air').

Most importantly, do the push and retract motion as slowly as possible. The anus is a very sensitive tunnel.

Absorbing the chords: At this stage, we recommend using the middle finger. It is longer and stronger than the rest, which allows your partner to experience ultimate pleasure. Before beginning, it's best to gently massage the external anus area using circular, caressing movements and to create wet, warm 'rings' around the 'kitchenette.' This sensual strumming of the strings relaxes the area and prepares it for the next step: Slow penetration with gentle, but strong thrusts beyond the front of the rectum while the tip of the penetrating finger moves slightly.

After you've gotten deep inside, we recommend continuing with the internal massage of the anus with circular movements between the interior walls so that you feel the magical touch of the 'kitchenette' gate through the skin and gradually relax your partner. Just as with the licking action, we recommend that the strumming recipient ('kitchen owner'), who will certainly be soaked with a storm of senses by this point, does the pushing motion. This increases the friction between the penetrating finger and the anus walls, which increases and intensifies the pleasure.

The first time you penetrate a finger into the 'kitchenette,' your partner is likely to feel a small amount of pain, which can sometimes persist until the following day. In every instance, the symptoms that come from finishing the symphony (pain in the anal area, walking funny, the feeling that a broom is stuck exactly where it shouldn't be, etc.) will pass quickly. With time, these symptoms will disappear altogether. The gentler and more carefully you act, the bigger the post-symphony smile will be – along with a small song in your heart.

As they say: It's not over until the fat lady sings…

Stage Four: The more the merrier

After successfully penetrating a single finger a few times, it's time to invite additional guests to the 'party' and expand your circle on the way to *Fabio's* exciting entry into the action. At this point, you can carefully penetrate with the thumb or two other fingers (as long as the thumb isn't one of them since we don't want to make our partner pass out). Also, just as before, you must lubricate your fingers, penetrate gently and slowly, relax your partner and be sensitive to their reactions.

Stage Five: A little help from a Friend

This stage isn't necessary, but is very strongly recommended.

Anal vibrators can be found in every sex shop. This vibrator is smaller and thinner than a regular one; it is used for smooth, gentle anal penetration and also helps in getting to the man's G-Spot. (See description later on in this chapter).

The goal here is another gradual expansion of the anus, providing more, thorough pleasure for the partner, and preparation for the final, decisive stage.

*Important note: Before penetration with an anal vibrator make sure to lubricate it or spread special cream that will help it to slip in. And, as you did in earlier stages, penetrate carefully and gently with the utmost sensitivity to your partner's reactions. (Not yet with ongoing penetration and extraction).

Stage Six: Touchdown!

The long-awaited moment has arrived. This is the stage during which your main pioneer fully enters into the partner's back gate. The dividing walls were knocked down, the foreplay is over and relaxation activities are now behind you. Now it's just you and the narrow, much-desired heavenly gates.

Your partner successfully crossed the path. Now, you can and should admit well-lubricated *Fabio* into the party (according to the cautions indicated in the last paragraph). The act of penetrating *Fabio* into the anus should be gradual, slow and answer all of your partner's needs. If she's 'into it,' you can expect a fireworks; if she's still not ready, give her the time she needs. The more she trusts you, the shorter *Fabio's* road into the 'kitchenette' will be.

Most important: During the act of anal sex, condoms must be used as the chances of contracting STDs – including AIDS, are particularly high.

Did you know?

Contracting and releasing the anus muscles during anal penetration doubles and triples the man's enjoyment and helps him finish faster…

Fingering

We highly recommend fingering your partner during anal sex (at each of the stages: one finger, two, and finally – Fabio himself). This increases sexual pleasure and arousal. However, not every position enables simultaneous fingering, and not every cook is a chef with coordination as impressive as our Maestro. Therefore, friends who still haven't mastered the bible completely should recommend that their partner masturbate on their own during penetration into the 'kitchenette.'

An additional recommendation for particularly open and liberated couples: During anal sex, your partner can work simultaneously on *Angelina* and her clitoris using a vibrator. The combination of anal and vaginal penetration and 'clitoral treatment' will give her a remarkable, multi-sensory explosion.

Suggested positions

Suit your position choices to experience level, comfort and collective needs of the two partners. And now, put on your chef's hat and hit the road!

Spooning

Spooning is highly recommended – especially for the beginners among us.

Penetration is performed as the female partner lies on her side with her partner lying on his side behind her, his stomach up against the woman's back. The woman folds her legs slightly toward her stomach, legs against one another, and her partner slowly and gently penetrates from behind.

Spooning is good for beginners, as the penetration is partial and does not enable the male partner to penetrate too quickly. Also, this unique position does enable him to finger the partner at the same time, and assists the 'naked chef' to better sense his 'penetrated' partner, and 'spoon feed her' as per her needs (too quickly, too hard, too slow, too much, etc.).

Doggie Style

The 'Doggie Style' position – looks exactly like it sounds. The female is on all fours (leaning on her hands with her knees resting on the floor) and the male, up against her behind, penetrates into her anus. Doggie Style is recommended mostly for the experienced chefs among us. It enables very deep, satisfying penetration for both partners, maneuvering space both for the maestro's hips and his wonder fingers, and gives his partner the ability to masturbate simultaneously without too much effort.

On the Stomach

In this position, the partner penetrates into the 'kitchenette' as his partner lies on her stomach, with a pillow resting between her hips and the bed raising the 'field of action.' Her legs are spread wide and the maestro, whose stomach is directly above her back, penetrates deeply and smoothly between them.

On the Stomach is especially effective for deep, smooth and thorough penetration. It also relieves both partners' hands since they are free throughout and it doesn't require motor genius or the 'octopus effect,' as I love to call it...

The Missionary Position

A well-known position familiar to us all. The penetration is with the female partner lying on her back with legs spread, a pillow resting under her hips, which she lifts up slightly to expose the anus. Her partner, facing her, leans in and 'squeezes' through her spread legs; he penetrates into her 'kitchenette' using this classic intercourse position.

The missionary position is particularly recommended for intimate lovers, since the partners face one another and their hands are free to hug, caress and kiss throughout the penetration.

The Contortionist

This position is similar to the Missionary position, with one small difference – the woman's legs are raised slightly toward her face, or can rest on the man's shoulders. The advantage of this position is that it enables total – and much easier – penetration by the culinary conqueror since the 'kitchenette' is higher up and more accessible than in the Missionary Position.

The Cowgirl

In this position, penetration occurs with the man lying on his back as the woman sits on top of his obtruding 'saddle.'

Regular Cowgirl: The naked chef penetrates his partner's 'kitchenette' while she faces him and sits on top of *Fabio*.

Reverse Cowgirl: The naked chef penetrates his partner's 'kitchenette' as she sits on *Fabio* backwards, with her back turned toward his face.

The advantages of the Cowgirl position is that it gives the woman control over the speed and depth of *Fabio's* penetration. This enables the wild cowgirl to rotate her hips (we recommend doing this gently – the rodeo yard is already very crowded) and makes it easier for the maestro to finger his rider, or for the wild cowgirl to masturbate on her own. There's no need for us to point out that just as with penetration into *Angelina*, there are an infinite number of positions for delving into the 'kitchenette.' Definitely let your imagination run wild and discover new methods for drilling in the constant chase after oil.

The Male G-spot

The male G-spot is located deep inside his 'kitchenette.' (When you insert the pad of your finger, it should be fully swallowed until the very end). If you want to give your Maestro a wonderful, dizzying orgasm that will make him come like a loud, exhilarating symphony, all you have to do is go down on him or work his gifted *Fabio* with your hand and simultaneously rub the naughty prostate.

Your loyal friend can't give you a precise, scientific explanation for what happens. But, who cares?! It works! And now on to conducting your symphony…

Kneel between the man's open legs while facing him, and gently penetrate your fingers about five or six centimeters into his 'kitchenette.' (Again, be sure to use rules of caution that you learned before).

When you get to the 'desired destination,' do the 'Come here' motion with your penetrating finger. (You shouldn't use the thumb the first time). The palm of your hand should be facing the man's stomach as the pad of the penetrating finger lovingly rubs against the excited spot. Simultaneously, 'spoil' curiously protruding *Fabio* with your warm tongue or other hand (just like you learned in 'Nice Rubbing' and 'The King's Pool').

Another position that requires a lot of female coordination: Penetrate your finger into the 'desired destination' while *Fabio* visits *Angelina* in the Cowgirl Position described in the last section.

It is important to note that most men enjoy and even become

addicted to this the minute they're exposed to it. Still, there are those that find it to be annoying and 'invasive.'

And finally... a mole in the pantry

To diversify and refresh anal sex, you can penetrate objects of different sizes and shapes into the 'kitchenette.' You need to make sure that they are smooth – so that they'll penetrate easily into the warm suitcase, and unbreakable – so that they won't break or come apart inside the 'kitchenette,' which would end your adventure in the emergency room. Well-informed sources tell stories about special hospital departments, whose purpose – among other things, is to find naughty moles who got lost inside the 'pantry.'

Aside from vibrators of different sizes and lengths, there is a highly recommended mole called 'Anal Beads.' This is an accessory made up of a strong rope with beads strung on it. The idea is to penetrate the beads into your partner's anus during sex and take it out (either at once or gradually, as per your partner's preference) a second before climax. Pulling out the beads intensifies the orgasm, bringing it to new heights with the combination of simultaneously pleasuring the 'engine' and the 'back burner.'

Anal beads are recommended for single use, as they tend to develop the 'chameleon effect.' They go in white (or red, yellow or blue) and come out brown and steaming hot...

Important note: After you've penetrated your partner's 'kitchenette' with *Fabio*, a finger, or any other type of mole, wash it well before a royal visit to *Angelina's* leaky house. This will prevent infection or inflammation that can confine little *Katie* to her bed...

Chapter 5

Just before it's over: Delay your climax

Almost every guy has experienced the embarrassing phenomenon of the 'sauce' taking preventative measures, otherwise known as: early ejaculation.

This usually happens when you've wanted a certain Marilyn for a long time, or a really long time has passed since your *Fabio* has gotten to know anything other than your loyal, supportive right hand.

You prepare for a festive moment, your *Marilyn* lies expectantly on the bed, but then, before she's gotten a word out, she starts to feel the warm, erupting sauce inside her *Angelina* or, if you decided to start 'slow,' on her hand.

You women probably also have experience with this bitter disappointment.

You're excited for 'bada-bing-bada-boom' with the man of your dreams – you put on make-up, make yourself look pretty, get dressed and then take your clothes off. Things start to shift gears, but then, instead of hot, long-lasting sex that reminds you of an expensive, three-course meal, you get a hastily-prepared tiny dessert.

Men: Don't be embarrassed, you are not alone in this battle. This happens to everyone, even to the best of 'em. It's a completely psychological issue that has no connection to your ability to function sexually. Your body, which hasn't been sexually active for a while, or got very excited from the desirable *Marilyn,* speeds up its activity and causes the 'sauce' to come out before its time.

Women: We ask for a bit of patience from the prima-donnas. Take into account that the amount of time it takes you to come is almost always longer than for the man. This is also a completely psychological issue. Aside from very few women who can come within a few seconds and up to a minute, most women need a respectable amount of 'action time' until they begin to hear victory bells and fanfares.

Another important 'hot item' to note is *Angelina's* high temperature and her narrow, tight-fitting cloak that 'closes' around *Fabio* and doesn't give him any other choice than to come before she does.

In this chapter we'll present you with two unique methods that will enable frustrated men to significantly delay coming and leave the 'sauce' in the nest until the right moment. We'll teach you how to climax after your *Marilyn,* pleasure her for long, extended periods and become the 'man of the hour' among your partner and her friends, who will certainly be very curious to hear about the 'New Kid on the Block.' You've already been told that word of mouth is the most effective and credible publicity there is, no?

And you'll think about her day and night

Below you will find two techniques plus a dirty trick that will turn your sexual abilities into something everyone's gossiping about…

The Great Wall of China

General

This wonderful method originates in Ancient China. It was created by Chinese experts whose power is in their ancient and thorough understanding of nature, and in particular, of the human body and human race.

This is an excellent, simple method for operation whose purpose is to stop the emission of sperm a few seconds before you come without sabotaging the imminent orgasm or the functioning of your 'active barrel' later on. After 'combat training' alone, you can also apply this wonderful method in the important battle against *Marilyn.*

Operating Instructions

If you place a mirror in front of your crotch, you will discover a pipe-like bump between your testicles and anus, which swells up when naughty *Fabio* is erect.

All you have to do during the training stage (and later, during the battle itself) is to get *Fabio* 'lifted,' notice the aforementioned swollen bump, and continue pleasuring *Fabio*. Then, about five seconds before you come (and no less!) – push on both sides of the tube using your finger and thumb.

Try to imagine that you are stopping the flow of your unruly garden hose. The pressure is meant to be very strong, but not so strong that it hurts. We just want to help the 'sauce' return home peacefully.

A similar, and no less effective, technique is to stop the 'sauce' by putting steady, decisive pressure on the bump using two or three of your middle fingers (meaning, index, middle and ring fingers) up against one another.

As a result of the intensive pressure, you will experience climax in every way, with the exception of one small thing – the sperm. Your pleasure is not affected (unless you focus on stopping the sperm and not on your fantastic orgasm). And if you watch *Fabio,* you'll notice that he jumps exactly like he does during a regular ejaculation.

This means: You won the Cowboy lotto! Your penis stayed erect even after his amazing finish (after which more will follow because of the 'friend brings a friend' network). Now you can continue and enjoy *Marilyn;* aside from the fact that *Fabio* didn't discharge any sperm, it will be business as usual.

The physical effect

The act of pressing your thumb and forefinger on the 'canal' stops the flow of sperm from the testicles toward the 'exit' from the penis. So basically, you're the only one that knows you came. There is no way *Marilyn* will assume the 'sauce' almost escaped; you can keep going and publicize *Fabio's* amazing talents, as if you were a 'Spitfire' plane with a 'wonder engine' and rust-proof steel able to fight for hours on end.

A small bonus on the side

Finally, we're equal. After years of suffering and 'operation anxiety,' we can also fake orgasms, but in exactly the opposite way. Women don't come but let us think that they have; we can come again and again while allowing them to think that we're not even close.

Keeping the good taste in your mouth

After 'pushing on the canal', our 'sauce' was an obedient soldier and didn't break out. Still, it's possible that after it passed through the testicle barrier, some of the sperm stayed in the tube of the penis. In this case, if *Marilyn* volunteers to give Fabio 'mouth-to-tube' resuscitation, she's likely to notice a bit of sperm in her mouth.

The Indian clerk

General

As is true with the best Indian traditions, this technique is based on the incredible power of thought. Yes, dear men, whether you believe in it or not, through the strength of your thought alone, you can achieve hours of penetration. That's right, hours! Your amigo here wouldn't joke. All of this is the fruit of research studies and the testimonies of loyal friends who tried the amazing theory on 'their meat'...

You don't have to use your hands, drugs or any chemicals. It is all the fruit of determination and thought. We won't pretend to be magician Uri Geller and bend spoons, but we keep them endlessly standing and erect.

The method being referred to requires a lot of patience and determination. Much like the previous method, it includes 'field training' on your own (which can last months) until a breakthrough with your current sweetheart. It is definitely worthwhile, gentlemen; this investment will yield particularly impressive profits.

The following short story is meant to help you in acknowledging the power of diligence and persistence, and in the case of the recounted story, about the power to earn a lot of money. (And to all those jumping up, we recommend reading through to the end. It isn't what you think.) 'A man was walking down the street, when suddenly, he noticed a half shekel resting on the sidewalk. He thought and thought, and finally decided to invest his small treasure in a big, juicy apple. But, the apple was a bit dusty. The man cleaned it off with his shirt sleeve. He shined, polished it, and then sold it for one shekel. With this shekel, the man bought two apples, cleaned them and sold them for two shekels exactly. With the two shekels that he earned, our shrewd merchant bought four apples and sold them for eight shekels. The smart, persistent man continued and continued until finally, he had accumulated enough money to open an apple store. He always cleaned the apples with his seasoned sleeve, sold more and more of them, until he had saved enough money to open another store.

He continued and continued like this, until one day, he gathered together his family members and gave them an impressive inheritance of twenty million dollars.'

The moral of this story: perseverance and determination will lead you to distant territory. They will change your life and allow additional doors to open for you.

Your determination is so powerful that nothing can stop it, even destiny!

A few words about Tantra

Tantra is a broad, ancient Indian doctrine that deals with a wide variety of issues in human life and enables its believers to improve their physical and spiritual lives beyond recognition. The West tends to mistakenly relate to it as a 'Sex Doctrine', as if it is the Kama Sutra's step-sister, but really, it's much broader and more interesting.

The Tantra does deal with sex, but it does so in terms of sexual energy, which serves as a basis for uplifting the soul and strengthening a person's spiritually. Tantra followers claim that 'advanced tantric practitioners' have the power to do real magic – to bless or curse others with magic that takes no time to come to fruition.

In this chapter, we'll present to you one of the Tantric methods for postponing or increasing the amount of time it takes the man to come.

The chapter is intended for both men and women, since women can also achieve an hour-long (or more) orgasm through 'Tantric training.' From here on in, dear women, even if the chapter is directed mainly at men, you can also complete the exhausting training course yourselves, assuming you want to turn your orgasm into something that is truly felt.

That's right. No more short dizzy spell, but instead the experience of ongoing flying that would cause even Supergirl to look bulky and lacking the ability to fly.

Important note

'The Tantric Training' is tiring and lasts for an extended period of time. It isn't intended for people with a weak character or 'short fuse.' It requires a lot of patience, steely determination and infinite perseverance.

Fitness Examination

If you belong to the group of people who prefer 'cutting corners' with a sandwich instead of eating a good, nutritious meal – it's best for you to skip to the next chapter.

If you're a member of the population for whom cooking a simple hamburger turns into a complicated culinary effort, then you should continue reading.

This unique technique has no shortcuts, no cheating and no 'cheat sheets.' There is no path other than the 'Yellow Brick Road' that sends Dorothy straight to seventh heaven.

So, take your time and expect hard, long-term and strenuous work that will bear fruit, but will also hurt a bit sometimes. And now, following all the introductions, the decision to continue reading this chapter is up to you, and only you.

The roots of the 'trunk'

If you've reached this paragraph, it means that either you belong to the second group or that this subject interests you enough to try. Either way, we wish you good luck.

And now back to the roots: According to the Tantra, your sperm is the energy of life. This energy is limited, meaning that each of you has a certain amount of energy that can never be renewed. Basically, the Tantra believes that the minute you finish up the energy that was given to you, you are meant to die (not so nice, is it?).

From this, we understand it is very important to preserve your sperm, and consequently, to avoid 'irresponsible ejaculation.' The Tantra suggests that you be very selective and seriously consider when to waste your life's energy and when to hold onto it for a rainy day.

Aside from these fatal consequences, the Tantra sees wasting sexual energy as the main cause of deterioration of man. It claims that the 'blind waste' of sperm keeps you, small mischievous ones, from living to your peak. Meaning, over-ejaculation of sperm causes misuse of your life energy, much like what happens with an uncovered pressure cooker or a marathon run on rocky ground.

I, your experienced friend, took into account that this approach will be perceived by most men as strange and unsubstantiated. This is due to the simple fact that a roaring lion – much like modern man – will have trouble perceiving his ejaculation as anything but the center of the universe, the evolutionary cause for human existence, or the source of the hole in the ozone layer and melted icebergs in the North Pole. Also, because man perceives his ejaculation as something that causes supreme pleasure, he is unable to see it as responsible for shortening his life expectancy.

This is a big mistake, gentlemen!

Only after trying the 'Great Wall of China' technique described in the beginning of this chapter, will you understand that the greatly admired ejaculation comes after climax and is actually just a psychological expression. The thick, whitish solution is all-in-all just the body's last signal to show that it experienced its dizzying height of pleasure. The whitish solution has no connection to your pleasure; you can 'celebrate' wonderfully without it. Therefore, according to the Tantra, the more you 'celebrate' without it, the more parties will be left in your lifelong calendar. Also, you will discover that you can extend an orgasm from just a few 'uplifting' seconds for your soul and genitals into a wonderful eternity of unlimited pleasure.

Sound strange and illogical? That's a sign that you're still thinking in a 'worldly' and not 'tantric' mindset.

Open your window, and take out the dividers and barriers. Prepare yourselves for an exciting journey of discovery.

Important note

You have to go through the training course alone; however, there is a stage at which you will need to add a partner so that you can practice as a team. As they say: 'Two heads are better than one.' Either way, when you get to party time, you'll celebrate together;

in the meantime, why not start with the less easygoing stage now?

To all the lone wolves out there

Not having a partner doesn't have to discourage you. In fact, exactly the opposite! The more diligently you practice, the more you'll become a 'skilled professional' and the demand for you on the market will continue to grow… who knows, maybe you'll suddenly inherit a harem of women from some deceased family member, just like in the best Tantric mythologies…

To all my courageous volunteers, I say to you: What's difficult in training is easy in battle!

The 'Point of No Return'

Before we start the training, a short, but extremely important explanation about the biological process that characterizes the male sex: The process of having sexual intercourse for you, Viking warriors, which is too short for your taste, features a specific point – a well-known biological moment – after which it's impossible to stop the ejaculation.

If we were to graph the process of sexual intercourse from the start until the climax, this is what it would look:

a The first stage in which erect *Fabio* begins to do his delightful work.
b The stage in which *Fabio* begins to warm up and becomes consistently firmer.
c *Fabio* has gotten in over his head in the private battle and begins to move toward the anticipated climax.
d The critical stage in which *Fabio* and the tension created by his bubbling sperm can no longer be stopped from launching all over the place.

The three points A, B and C represent stages during which you can do a U-turn, and stop naughty *Fabio*. The only point at which *Fabio* and his bubbling friends are like a rocket already launched off the base and never to return is Point D, otherwise known by its professional name: The Point of No Return. Chronologically, this point (or P.N.R.) happens in the half second before you come. Until this decisive moment, you can use various means to stop the 'sauce' from breaking out. Afterwards, you can't, dear fighters, do anything to stop either your orgasm or your explosive emission. The point of no return is an important moment in the tantric system, and we'll work on it later in this chapter.

Operating Instructions

The strenuous training process for 'erecting an almost eternal wall' can be done either by yourself or together with your partner. The goal at this initial stage is to come (enjoy it, Cowboy, as we'll get to the stages in which you'll be spared this too). You must do it slowly, so that you can imagine and feel every stage of the graph, up until the point of no return. Therefore, you should touch *Fabio* as gently as possible, leading him peacefully to the anticipated point. If you do this as a twosome, the responsibility to slowly, orally pleasure *Fabio* falls on you, *Marilyn* (see the 'King's Pool'), or give him a slow, smooth hand-job (see 'Nice Rubbing').

After you've arrived at the point of no return, it's important that you fully feel it and learn that feeling well. At this stage, the Tantric experts ask you to remember how many contractions there were as you landed *Fabio's* plane – in the area below the balls (found inside the body). There are fighters that report experiencing a number of contractions, and there are those who report just one. There are no clear, unequivocal rules about this number. So, for the sake of becoming acquainted with your 'orgasmic system,' remember how many contractions you experienced.

To avoid confusion, you should count just the number of contractions you experienced from the 'point of no return' through to the ejaculation, not including any contractions you experienced during the emission itself. The 'point of no return' is the critical stage on which you are working, and not the ejaculation – that's what we're trying to delay.

Did you come? Relax, enjoy and rest on your laurels until tomorrow – then your real training begins.

For whom the bell tolls

The goal of this training is to make sure that when the wonderful bells of orgasm toll, they ring for your happy partner, and not you! Until you finish the exhausting training, your *Fabio* will be so seasoned and 'worn out' that he will be able to lead sensual *Marilyn* from orgasm to orgasm through many, long hours until finally, he hears the delightful sound of orgasm bells ringing in his ears. If you are really interested in having this happen, then go on, get to work!

Now you've arrived at the second stage, the slightly more difficult stage of the training process: If you are together, then begin having slow, gentle sex. If you are relying on your loyal hand alone, then stroke *Fabio* as gently as possible. In either case, the goal is to enjoy, take your time and envision the graph throughout. At some point, you will internalize the graph and know by yourself which stage you're at in relation to the point of no return.

When you're really close to the point of no return, stop! Tighten the reins on the galloping horse's neck and do not, under any circumstances, continue touching erect *Fabio,* no matter how much he begs.

Now stop yourself, calm down and allow *Fabio* to rest from his feverish activity.

At the same time, count the number of contractions you experienced at the point of no return and remember it.

Are you calm? Start the process over with the slow, gentle activity that you were asked to do at the beginning, and again this time, stop about half a second before you reach the point of no return.

I know it's tough, amigos, and you really want to shake me upside down right now, but there's nothing you can do about it. You committed to an exhausting training program. Do you want to turn into roaring tigers? Do you want *Fabio* to make Superman look like Little Red Riding Hood's lost sister? So then, just like the dance instructor in Fame says: 'You have to pay to achieve fame!' Your *Fabio* definitely knows what she means right now. Now that you've stopped excited *Fabio*, count the number of contractions you experienced at the point of no return and remember it. That's it for tonight, my courageous soldiers, you've passed the first stage and you were great! All you have left to do is smile proudly, go to sleep and get a good night's rest before tomorrow's training. Have a restful night...

Another dangerous training day

Good morning friends! Again today you can expect a routine that is not simple, with one difference: You already know the trick and come to training more courageous and a bit more experienced than before...

Just like yesterday, today you will also have intercourse (or work with your trusty hand) to the familiar point of no return. After you've reached it, stop and count the number of contractions you experienced. The goal of this training is to continually increase the number of contractions you have before reaching the point of no return.

It's important to note that there's a high amount of pleasure during the contractions, and so you should try to experience it completely while making sure you don't come!!! If you miss one time, the unfortunate breakthrough means that you have to begin your difficult training course over from the beginning to get your body used to postponing orgasms from the start. So, be strong, pat yourselves on the back, and even if you have the neurotic need to excel at everything – this time, don't finish what you started.

Food for the road

This may seem simple and easy, but now we are getting to the small trap. You have to continue doing what you did yesterday and today for between three and six months.

You heard correctly – six months. Does it sound like a lot? But really, what is six months when compared to an eternity of wild, dizzying sex, a *Fabio* who functions like the Duracell bunny, and satisfied, gossipy women who don't hesitate to talk about the new 'meteor' in their life with every acquaintance they can?

You'll enjoy like you've never enjoyed before, your partner will finally succeed in coming, and the line outside your house will look like the cats in heat who wait for Spitz – my naughty, horny cat.

Promotion Ceremony

Congratulations! You've successfully completed your exhausting journey. Now you deserve the rank of 'great fuck' and master in slow, continuous pleasure.

This is the stage at which you are apparently skilled enough, at least as much as mischievous Spitz, as demonstrated by long contractions lasting a few minutes (as opposed to the two short contractions you had at the beginning), an orgasm that goes on and on, and exciting, arousing sex that ends only when you've decided the time has come to air out the sheets.

Did you know?

The Chinese believe that if a man succeeds in making a woman come ten times consecutively during one round of sexual intercourse (regardless of technique: penetration, going down on her, or fingering), they've established eternal life together. Your trusty friend isn't sure that eternal life is your secret wish – but the reputation for having an especially long shelf life will certainly make every man on the planet happy.

A few small splinters on the 'King's Path'

Testicle Pain

Yes, it happens. If the persistent, loyal 'fighter' doesn't finish for a long time, or alternatively, he stimulates *Fabio* but doesn't allow him to come satisfactorily, he's likely to feel a pain in his lower stomach, in the area above his 'artillery tube'.

A small secret for you ladies: If you stimulated little *Katie* and didn't allow her to climax, this can also cause pain in the lower abdominal area, right above *Angelina*. We're not making this up; this is testimony from various women who dared to share the secrets of their Norwegian princess with me.

It's important to clarify that this information is not meant to be used as a justification to do anything your partner asks (he can always go to a private corner and ease the pain 'by hand'), but you should know that the balls do have difficult labor pains as well; it's not just the chickens. In short, 'Viking warriors' should take into account that testicle pain is likely to be part of the complicated process of moving toward Tantric happiness. This will continue for a while, but, the more you practice, the faster it will pass.

The quiet dissemination

During the training period, as you avoid ejaculating more sperm, a less pleasant after-effect will accompany you: the smell of sperm in your sweat. Since the sperm accumulates and doesn't find its way out like it normally does, it instead evaporates from the body through alternative methods. It's not so pleasant, but a small price to pay for the final outcome. One potential solution for this problem is drinking a lot of water. You can dilute your sweat and its smell.

There are rumors that some women are still able to smell sperm in the man's sweat. Maybe this is true, maybe not – but either way, you have a few good months to check and to get back to us with an answer...

'Dirty' trick

General

This trick is meant for all the smart 'Cowboys' who use condoms.

This is the opportunity for your devoted educator to give you a piece of moral advice and emphasize that the use of condoms is recommended and vital for all those who have occasional sex, or whose partner has yet to have an AIDs or STD test.

Operating Instructions

For those new to the field, condoms come in twelve-packs.

All you have to do is take a new condom from the pack and to make a small hole at the end of its wrapper, at the very corner – without hurting the condom itself. (It's very important to make sure that your hole missed the condom). Leave the box somewhere on the side and wait about a month or two without opening it.

During this time, the condom has enough time to dry out (due to the small hole that you pierced) and now it's ready for 'action.' Put it on *Fabio* and go out to play.

The big bonus

Basically, when the dry, brittle condom is on *Fabio,* it serves as a heat separator between him and smoking *Angelina,* which enables our 'Rocket boy' to continue pleasing her without being influenced by her abundant heat and moisture. This effective divider promises a big and significant delay before impatient

Fabio's ejaculation; he is even able to provide his partner with absolute pleasure.

You, ladies, shouldn't feel any difference. The feeling is the same quick, repetitive one of kisses between Fabio and *Angelina*.

What smells more: your 'Lakarda' or the trick?

This trick is slightly smelly, but, ladies, it preserves the option for us to increase *Fabio's* functioning time by self perforation of the condom. When your 'cobra,' like always, asks to give you a short, fast 'bite', instead, give him the condom and make sure the 'bite' is long and satisfying. He won't always love the idea, since every man wants to enjoy what nature gave him, but in the end, he'll accept your ruling. He'll give his *Fabio* a long-term lesson in patience, and you'll win a wonderful, fantastic experience.

Splinters on the 'Queen's Path'

This trick is slightly dangerous, since there is a chance that you'll miss the hole, and you and your 'cobra' will get a perforated, unsafe condom.

Additionally, it's best that you don't wait too long with the 'treated condom.' That creates a danger that the condom will dry out and rip during sex – and then you'll be exposed to both STDs and unwanted pregnancy.

Important note

This recommendation is offered without any author responsibility. You should consider the danger that comes from the use of any old condom.

In a hurry

To all those impatient people who insist on a 'waiting period' until the condom has dried out, we recommend putting holes in a few packs at once, and then enjoying regular – even daily, sex with one 'treated condom' for each day.**A small trick with a few**

whitish stains: For anyone who prefers the shorter method that requires less 'investment,' we recommend allowing *Fabio* to come before his date with *Marilyn.* If you masturbate a bit before sex, I can promise you that the 'whitish tension' will take longer the second time and promise *Angelina* longer, more satisfying pleasure. Who knows? Maybe you'll even hear the bells ring together tonight.

Chapter 6

Body Heat: The Missionary Position and other sex positions

A few opening shots

In this short, abridged chapter, we'll present you with the crème de la crème of the wide world of positions.

As you probably already know, and have even experienced on your own body, each person has their favorite position – whether because of age, the different anatomical structures of *Jessica* and *Rabbit*, or due to the many odd and different reasons that make one person prefer strawberry, another banana and a third walnuts.

There are many, many positions on the planet but, in one chapter that would be exhausting and boring, mostly because you can see them in books, movies and websites.

Therefore, friends, we've collected just the 'elite' positions for you, which also supplies a short, easy-to-read chapter for all the lazy people out there…

Two important milestones

So that *Fabio's* visit with gentle *Angelina* goes smoothly and painlessly, keep in mind that all advice received up until now in earlier chapters should be applied to the royal visit (penetration). Our purpose is to enable *Angelina* to get a little wet, thus making penetration into the magical crevice easier. As you remember, the way to get *Angelina* wet is to stimulate and pleasure her.

Also, remember the first penetration must be gentle and slow, so that you don't hurt *Jessica*. Later down the road, you should increase the speed and intensity, but always – of course – while paying attention to her reactions.

The finish line

As you already learned in the chapters on 'Nice Rubbing' and the 'King's Pool,' in most cases *Jessica* will climax by rubbing her clitoris and/or G-spot. Very few of our female friends will require work on the rest of the 'Me'arat haMachpela' to experience the anticipated climax (what's called a vaginal orgasm). Whereas our naughty *Rabbits* – ok, it's no secret that the narrower, warmer and wetter the vagina, the faster the 'weapon collapse' will be.

And now, onto the positions themselves:

On the Stomach

In this position, *Fabio* penetrates into *Angelina* as *Jessica* lies on her stomach with legs spread wide. The partner's stomach is located on *Jessica's* back, and following the first penetration, she closes her legs, so that her partner's legs surround hers on the right and left.

In this wonderful position, *Rabbit's* and *Jessica's* orgasms will be quick, strong and powerful, even though the penetration itself is not particularly deep.

Rabbit's climax is quick because the penetration is dense and tight; and for *Jessica* – this position enables her partner to pleasure *Angelina*'s 'Miracle button' with his hand during penetration (see 'Nice Rubbing').

Missionary Position taken up a notch

In this position, *Jessica* lies on her back, legs spread, and *Rabbit* lies on top of her, so that his stomach is on top of hers. Until now it's entirely missionary, right? Now we're coming to the upgrade.

If *Rabbit* wants to enhance the position, he should lean on his elbows and lift his butt upward, so that *Fabio* penetrates *Angelina* at a vertical angle.

Basically, in this position, flexible *Fabio* is at an angle of almost ninety degrees from *Rabbit's* body.

The upgraded penetration creates a pleasure-filled friction with *Jessie's* 'Miracle Button', which gives your precious maiden great satisfaction, and also greatly pleases your dear *Fabio*. However, naughty one, this position might tire you out relatively quickly, as you are working both the hand and hip muscles.

Doggie Style

The Doggie Style position is exactly like its name sounds. Penetration in this position is done when *Jessica* bends down on all four (hands and knees resting on the floor) and the *Rabbit* is up against her from behind, penetrating *Fabio* into the magical kingdom.

This position is highly recommended, as it allows deep, satisfying penetration for both *Rabbit* and *Jessica* – and, at the same time as *Fabio* works on her G-spot, he can also pleasure her 'Miracle Button' by hand ('Rosh HaNikra' style).

Important note: Since this position provides deep, thorough penetration, the act of penetrating must start slowly and carefully. Intensity and speed should only increase later on, and continue until *Jessica* signifies that it no longer feels good and has begun to hurt. *Rabbit*, take into account that many women find deep penetration to be painful. Therefore, be attentive to your partner's needs, it will pay off on Judgment Day. (Just ask *Fabio*, he can tell you…)

Cowgirl

The penetration in this position is done as *Rabbit* lies on his back with *Jessica* sitting on his protruding 'saddle.'

Face-to-Face

This time, *Fabio*, the crowd favorite, visits *Angelina*'s deep territories as our *Jessica* sits on top of him, facing *Rabbit's* happy face.

Reverse Cowgirl

In this position, *Fabio* visits noble *Angelina* while *Jessie* sits on top of him – but with her back facing *Rabbit's* face.

The Cowgirl positions work on the G-spot of *Jessica's* clitoris, depending of course on the angle at which she moves on top of *Fabio*. Given our deep connection, I will assume, rebellious sisters, that you can find these two magical spots on your own.

This position is recommended for women in general, and in particular, for the virgins among us because we are the ones to set the speed and intensity of penetration.

A mixed blessing

This position doesn't always pleasure the *Rabbit* to the same degree, since not every angle of penetration is comfortable and suited to *Fabio's* sensitive structure. Our Galilean prince's angle is usually between 30-40 degrees toward *Rabbit's* stomach; so that you don't torment your partner too much, you should do the up and down motion on top of *Fabio* at this angle. (*Jessica* shouldn't be sitting on the testicles, but further in, closer to *Rabbit's* face).

If you prefer to be a bit selfish – something that is legitimate on occasion (as long as you don't go overboard), you can ignore the *Rabbit's* preferences and move up and down at the angle most comfortable for you. (No need for concern. This doesn't really hurt him, unless you go wild and 'ride' *Fabio* at an expressly impossible angle).

This also provides another benefit, my dears: Because of the *Rabbit's* discomfort from the 'angle' problem described above, he will come slower. *Jessicas* whose partners just finished the excellent training in the chapter, 'Berla, Berla don't move,' can expect a big bonus.

So, how do they say it out West? 'Onward!'

Trouble on the way to Heaven

In most cases, the 'Me'arat HaMachpela' fits *Fabio's* size. However, in cases where our *Fabio* is particularly big and wide, penetration will be difficult for gentle *Angelina*. For this reason, in every instance and regardless of *Fabio's* size, two things are essential:

Angelina should be wet and lubricated before penetration.

Penetration must be slow and done gradually.

A Jessica who has not been visited by *Fabio* in a long time is likely to find that her 'Me'arat HaMachpela' has become a bit narrower… don't worry, that's completely natural. Your cave will widen and adapt to *Fabio's* size after your first round of sex.

Other causes of misfortune in the 'Me'arat haMachpela' are constriction from birth (women with a narrow vagina) or psychological pressure. In this case, *Jessica* should be relaxed (give her warmth, love, and foreplay). Penetrate slowly and carefully, but only after a few dates and other sexual activities with her.

For women with special anxiety, who don't relax with regular methods, I suggest going to a gynecologist and finding out if it's a medical problem. Also, if it's a psychological problem, you can go for counseling to outmaneuver the problem from the top and not 'down below.'

Usable for every situation

After effect

Sometimes, when the *Rabbit* puts *Fabio* inside *Angelina*, you might hear a fart sound that results from the release of air that entered the vagina during intercourse. Don't laugh at your *Jessica*. This could insult her. But also bear in mind that *Fabio* is no less responsible for the flatulence than *Angelina*. Please control yourself…

Lot's wife

If one of the partners reaches orgasm before the other (regardless of how), the second partner (who hasn't come yet) should stay in the same position without moving. *Angelina* and *Fabio* are very sensitive in the critical moment of coming, and any movement, small as it may be, is likely to sabotage the wonderful, orgasmic experience.

Stay at home

Dear Rabbit, if you climaxed, enjoy it all you can, but don't hurry to take *Fabio* out of *Angelina*'s 'Me'arat haMachpela.' Stay inside the warm, enveloping cave for a little while; this demonstrates intimacy, makes *Jessica* feel like you have a lot of patience and shows that you are definitely not a 'hit and run' guy. After a bit, you are responsible for using another one of the positions you learned in this chapter or 'leaving for a new campaign' completely (taken from another chapter in this book) and arousing the surprised *Jessica*.

This has to be said for once and for all

It's not the length that matters; it's the width.

A few small things to conclude

As we've already suggested more than once – use your imagination with positions, accessories and non-routine places to have sex. Do it at every angle and in every possible direction; mix in legs, feet, hands and tongue; add pillows, satin sheets; do it in your parents' house, in the plane bathroom, on kitchen chairs, on an inflatable boat in the water or in the lifeguard stand. And most importantly, use more than one position in every round of intercourse – unless the position and angle bring lots of pleasure and don't cause steamy *Jessica* or *Rabbit* any pain from the passion.

Wow, someone should turn on the air-conditioning or a fan – **it's hot in here...**

Chapter 7

Trifles to fill in the spaces: Add more spice in bed

Now, after we've covered all the truly important and significant topics, we won't send you on your 'adventurous' way until we've equipped you with a few colorful candies to decorate the rich cake that we've baked for you throughout the book. In this last, summarizing chapter, we've gathered small, effective tips that don't need enough details to fill an entire chapter, but definitely can enhance your sex life significantly.

The objective is all the gestures, positions, words and minutiae that are used to provide a small, naughty spark to light the fire between you and *Mister Big*, or you and *Miss Robinson*.

Firing up *Miss Robinson's* Engine

Just like toys

Foreplay is very important to *Miss Robinson*. Before getting to the main course, *Miss Robinson* loves to have her senses stimulated by appetizers that arouse and boost her appetite. So, before you get close to the 'unification' between *Fabio* and *Angelina*, please provide a lot of love and affection to the 'party's' other participants: mouth, tongue, breasts, stomach, buttocks, and anyone else in need of attention. This will flood *Angelina* with juicy nectar expectantly awaiting *Fabio's* visit.

Dirty Talk

Dear men, you should know that a few lust-filled words in the middle of a boring, routine day can dramatically bump up *Miss Robinson*'s impulse threshold. Whether you are standing right next to her, or you whisper a few words into the telephone –

sharing details of *Fabio's* naughty exploits inside her *Angelina,* here, now and unadulterated, can definitely get the job done. *Miss Robinson*'s hormones will jump sky high. And, when *Fabio* finally meets *Angelina,* you'll be sorry you didn't put acoustic walls up in the apartment.

Sweet to him, sweet to him

When you get to the very heart of the storm, take a piece of good advice from us for breaking the routine sex and 'sweetening the moment': Spreading maple syrup or chocolate sauce on *Angelina* will get you both hot and bothered. *Mister Big* will sensually lick your 'candy', and enjoy himself more and more as the syrup's sweetness gets diluted by the taste of little *Katie*. You, on the other hand, will experience an amazingly remarkable orgasm, as your partner will be unable to pull his tongue away from *Katie's* fire.

Closed for renovations

One of the most highly recommended exercises to increase sexual enjoyment – for both *Miss Robinson* and *Mr. Big* – is the Kegel Exercise. Its purpose is to strengthen *Miss Robinson's* lower vaginal muscles and improve her ability to contract *Angelina* during penetration. In this way, *Angelina*'s muscles will be contracted during *Fabio's* visit, and the friction will increase everyone's satisfaction level. All you have to do, *Miss Robinson,* is to begin practicing contracting the vaginal muscles, just like you do when you try to stop peeing.

Make sure to contract *Angelina* for three seconds (and afterwards release), nine times consecutively, to complete one 'training set.' Do the 'training set' three times a day, every day, for six weeks consecutively.

You're welcome to do the 'training set' anywhere. As long as you don't make funny faces while you contract, no one will know what is going on in your secret cave.

At the end of the training program, when Fabio comes for a 'visit to the homeland' with *Angelina*, every contraction like this will wonderfully raise both the level of your enjoyment and also that of *Mister Big*, as *Angelina*'s warm walls will skillfully tighten around him.

Did you know?

There are those who claim that men with developed '*Fabio* muscles' – after the Kegel Exercise – are able to stop their ejaculation without using their hands, just like the Chinese method mentioned in the 'Just before it's over.'

Firing up *Mr. Big's* Engine

The Naked Truth

A common myth (mostly in movies) is that we, men, 'melt' for revealing, sexy baby-doll dress, and that we want the 'arousing' piece of clothing to adorn *Miss Robinson*'s body every night. Unfortunately, ladies and gentlemen, I must admit that the real arousal comes from the thought that soon the baby-doll outfit will be removed and we can finally 'dance together.' The clothes themselves don't increase or take away from arousal; it's just a test before the real thing.

Organ rescue

If you really want to turn *Mister Big* on, try this trick. In the middle of the day and in a crowded place, move your hand down toward the covered area of his body. (Try, of course, to have no one else see you). The danger that someone is likely to see you treating his 'treasures' with a 'trusty hand' turns your partner on and makes him feel attractive, since *Miss Robinson* can't control herself and must touch him.

It's interesting to be interested in the same interest

The above tip does not start just with actions, but also with words. Just like women, men will also be very happy to receive a 'comprehensive description' in the middle of a crowded place of what naughty *Miss Robinson* would be interested in doing to them.

The more you use your wild imagination, the more 'fireworks' you'll see a few hours later.

Careful, danger of slipping

This wonderful advice was collected from Patpong Street in Bangkok. Women there really understand what can turn *Mister Big* on. (This isn't a wisecrack; they host *Fabio* in *Angelina*'s generous abode for a living).

The idea is to make your skin soft and lovely like silk by spreading a generous layer of body cream on your body and then adding a layer of talcum powder.

I promise you, *Miss Robinson,* your partner will be positive that he is hovering over cotton fields and will have trouble identifying your smooth, delightful and wonderful skin.

The Chest of Surprises – the Unisex booklet

Below are a few spicy pieces of advice, intended for both sexes. This tip collection can be used both for the experienced, romantic *Mr. Big* and for the seductive and sexy *Miss Robinson*. So, eat with pleasure, and remember: Only those who don't eat also don't need to gather crumbs from their apron.

Live and die from the tongue

If you want your partner to feel loved, attractive and respected during the sex, don't keep your thoughts to yourself. Declare your feelings out loud or in a sensual whisper into his/her ear.

Declarations about your partner's incredible body and each of their attractive organs (butt, chest, *Fabio, Angelina*) will be happily accepted, and will even increase their enjoyment and self-confidence. Of course you shouldn't stop there – because if you want to demonstrate to *Mr. Big* or *Miss Robinson* that this isn't just lip service – kiss, lick and suck that body part a number of times. Bon appetit!

Laughter on the side

As much as we've recommended you compliment your partner's body or performance, we also stress that never, under any circumstance, can you ridicule *Mr. Big* or *Miss Robinson*'s 'performance' or any part of their body. Men and women tend to be very sensitive and vulnerable about their bodies: being overweight, chest size, different smells, size and thickness of *Fabio*, etc. Did you know, for example, that when *Fabio* is exposed to cold or gets out of water, he shrinks and loses his original size? Just ask George Costanza; he'll tell you that *Fabio* also sometimes needs refuge… The same is true with *Mister Big* and *Miss Robinson*'s performance ability. Avoid sarcastic comments such as: too slow, too fast, clumsy, lies like a dead fish, etc. These things eat away at your partner's self-confidence and surely won't be helpful.

Diplomatic contact

One of the best ways to arouse your partner without actually saying the word sex is a massage. This wonderful touch decreases tension, loosens up tight muscles, and increases the hormone level (in preparation for the amazing sex that will come afterward) and creates intimacy. If you use this method once in a while, you'll find that your sex life improves incredibly.

The massage recommended for 'heating up the atmosphere' is a Swedish massage. (It is very common all over the world, and works with intimate body 'kneading'). It is gentle, nice and preferred over its friends in the professional massage world, including the Thai Massage – which most people find to be painful, the Indian Massage – which is pleasant but requires a lot of oil that dirties the 'work space,' the Chinese Massage – which isn't bad at all but can't be compared to the pure pleasure offered by its Swedish cousin.

Ballad to the bottle

If you both feel like 'losing your heads' and getting into a dazed, contented mood with your partner, then alcohol of any type (wine, beer or vodka) is what you need. A proportional flow of alcohol into the body just before a meal will ensure you have an unrestricted and liberated atmosphere, with decreased awkwardness and a break in the tension (non-sexual, of course) with *Mister Big* or *Miss Robinson*. It will also exponentially increase the degree of your sexual stimulation, and the sex... oh, this is sex you will remember for a very long time.

One, Two and Go

Communication, friends, communication! This is one of the most significant things in a relationship (and especially an intimate one) between two people. Your partners are not fortune tellers or palm readers, and if you want them to know how to pleasure you, you should begin learning to talk. This is a crystal-clear way to improve your sex life.

Tell them what feels nice, what turns you on the most, and what less so. Also fantasies, even the wildest ones, are definitely something you can – and should – share with your partner.

Drying the swamp

After the 'tango for two' has ended successfully and your partner lies 'like liquid' and full of sweat, we highly recommend wiping off and cooling her/him with a wet wipe (generally used for wiping a baby's bottom). Move it over their body, without missing any body part, and to finish, blow some cold air on the moist area. This is a fantastic pampering for *Mister Big* – who worked hard, or *Miss Robinson* – who also put her hands into the pie. They will certainly want to 'tango for two' again just for this wonderful enjoyment again later.

I'm all ears

It's a well-known fact that ears are a particularly tender and sensitive place – and so they also arouse like crazy. While building tension before the 'meeting of the greats' between *Fabio* and '*Angelina*,' gently blow into your partner's ear, lick inside it (using just a little bit of saliva) and tug lightly on their earlobes. This works like magic... your partner will lose control from enjoyment and sexual excitement.

The more advanced among you can 'work' simultaneously on the 'main guest' waiting in the Southern Wing, and guarantee that *Mister Big* or *Miss Robinson* will have the time of their life.

A Christmas-style surprise

In most sex stores, you can find a 'snowy' accessory, or more specifically, 'iceberg,' which looks like *Fabio's* twin brother. It is shaped like male genitalia. You pour water inside it and then put it immediately into the freezer. The result: an attractive, impressive *Fabio* made entirely out of ice.

Operating instructions:

Take the 'Frozen Fabio' out of the freezer and let it thaw for a few minutes. A fact of physics is that water doesn't tend to freeze in a uniform manner, and the 'frozen creations' flicker into the world with an abundance of tiny bumps. Using this creation is likely to injure and hurt *Angelina*, and quickly end what has just started.

After 'Frozen Fabio' has ended his waiting period, place him next to the bed and then, when you are in the height of the 'two person party' (fingers or tongue in a homeland visit with *Angelina*), surprise *Miss Robinson* and gently penetrate the frozen twin into *Angelina*.

Avoid forgetting the 'Frozen Lord' in *Angelina*'s dormitory. Our Norwegian princess is a bit sensitive, and ongoing touch with 'Frozen Fabio' will give her cold sores.

The most important thing is to not consecutively use the same 'Frozen Twin,' even if you made sure to give *Angelina* rest time. The hidden danger is that 'Frozen Fabio' (who continues to thaw) is likely to break inside *Angelina*'s caves and cause pointy, sharp pieces of ice to disperse deep into the 'Milky Way.' If this happens, it is very difficult to get 'Broken Fabio' out of his deep hiding places, and our little *Katie* will get cold sores in the meantime.

Conclusion: Use the 'Frozen Twin' when at its peak, and let the successful, 'human' brother do the rest of the work.

The final patches in *Mr. Big's* Suit

Deep intoxication

Now is the time to remind you, dear men, sometimes you are also allowed to lean back, close your eyes and enjoy what *Miss Robinson* has to offer.

Just as your little lady knows how to leave everything behind and invest in a fun nirvana when you pleasure her *Angelina*, you can also give her the same task.

When *Miss Robinson*'s long tongue decides to give wet, focused treatment and devoted care to *Fabio*, or when your woman turns into a 'rider' on the erect snake, we recommend that you focus on your personal enjoyment.

This is a moment to let go, close your eyes, forget about everything and enjoy as much as possible. Put your hands behind your neck, or in any other place that's comfortable for you, and try to avoid sending them toward *Angelina* or *Miss Robinson*'s breasts, even if that increases and intensifies your stimulation. Trust me, the meditation and concentration on *Miss Robinson*'s activity alone will enrich your pleasure immeasurably.

Now, after you've come, keep your eyes closed longer and find the pleasure through to the end. Don't start worrying about what your lady thinks, how she feels or what she expects you to do – just enjoy the last waves of your orgasm.

When you've relaxed completely, open your eyes, give *Miss Robinson* a big, loving smile and thank her wholeheartedly for the 'devoted care.' Don't forget, it's also important for *Miss Robinson* to know and feel that you enjoyed yourself. She will reach the stars when you moan excitedly, orgasm and discharge juicy 'nectar' from *Fabio's* head out of your body – and it's best if not onto her clean sheets.

The Emperor's New Clothes

Your 'erect' king's underwear is more and more of a significant issue today. Because of real life dangers – diseases passed during sex, sexually transmitted diseases, or even unwanted pregnancy that can lead to abortion and grief – you need to be on guard and to add *Mr. Hat* – the condom – into your everyday list of expenses. The condom has a huge significance; its quality is also very important. There are a number of companies on the market that supply good-quality, highly recommended condoms; there is even a list of FDA approved condoms, which is considered to be the strictest in its regulations. (It looks at condom thickness, elasticity, etc.).

Ladies! Don't trust your *Mister Big* to go and choose the highest quality condom, especially if you're dealing with an occasional partner who is more focused on his amazing sex than your safety. Purchase the appropriate 'cap' on your own, so that you'll always be equipped with effective, safe protection and not with a cheap condom destined for trouble.

One of the most important things about condoms is the way that *Fabio* puts them on.

As most of you probably already know, at the end of each condom there is a type of loose tip – a narrower addition of rubber, meant to absorb the sperm. When you put the cap on, don't stretch it too much and make sure to leave the tip loose and empty. The reason for this is that during sperm emission, a bubbly mass is added into the condom, intended to go peacefully from *Fabio's* 'exit opening' to the lose tip. If your Mr. Cap is stretched too tightly around *Fabio,* the mass and the stress created are likely to aggravate the condom and rip it.

The Trampoline Effect

If you're interested in charging up your sex life and 'jumping' it to an unprecedented level, then we have exactly what you're looking for. When you and *Miss Robinson* already feel very comfortable with each other, do 'Just like Toys' – after all, it is foreplay – and then 'check the wetness' of little *Angelina.* If the royal princess is wet enough, spread a handful of Pop Rocks on her. You will then see a vagina dancing the samba, with your very own eyes. Your *Angelina* will get into the rhythm, and the candies will 'make her lips and 'magic button' 'bounce.' It will be a sweet and lively experience for you both. *Miss Robinson,* for her part, is also invited to try this highly recommended technique. All she has to do is put a handful of Pop Rocks into her mouth and then dive toward *Mr. Big's* 'snorkel,' which will certainly be breathless after incredible pleasure…

Chapter 8

Go in Peace, the keys are all inside!

If you've gotten to this point and applied all of the advice we've given along the way, it seems that we are dealing with a qualified, very mischievous 'Sex Fiend'. You already know well how to drive *Mr. Big* or *Miss Robinson* crazy, both from the 'front' and the 'back.' *Fabio* and *Angelina* are your best friends; you understand that hands are meant for more than just picking your nose; your tongue is experienced in licking flavors other than strawberry-banana at the nearby ice cream parlor; and very soon, you will be able to give a lesson to the police on everything about 'Live Bombs.'

Assuming that the first read helped you get the basics, but before the 'Pied Piper of Hamelin's' capabilities have taken root in you (we do hope you'll be just like him in the end), this is the time to go back for a second read. That will help you to internalize the material learned and review thoroughly, until it becomes second nature – and it will, if you want it to!!

Now, after you've acquired the vital information and before you go tell every other person how to become a 'Sex Fiend' himself, take one last piece of advice from your Guardian Angels: Keep the cards close to your chest and leave the singing to Pavarotti and his friends. After all, you wouldn't want your ex's new boyfriend to give an equal performance just because he heard from someone, who heard from someone, who heard from someone about this book...

That's it friends – from here on in it's up to you.

We've put the keys to a prestigious, beautiful Jaguar into your hands. It's fast, sophisticated, beautiful, safe and intended to leave a long line of jealous people behind you... all that's left now is to move, straighten the mirrors and press hard on the gas pedal.

Go in peace, the keys are inside!

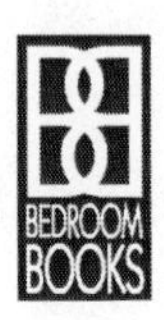

Romance, erotica, sensual or downright ballsy. When you want to escape: whether seeking a passionate fulfilment, a moment behind the bike sheds, a laugh with a chick-lit or a how-to – come into the Bedroom and take your pick. Bedroom readers are open-minded explorers knowing exactly what they like in their quest for pleasure, delight, thrills or knowledge.